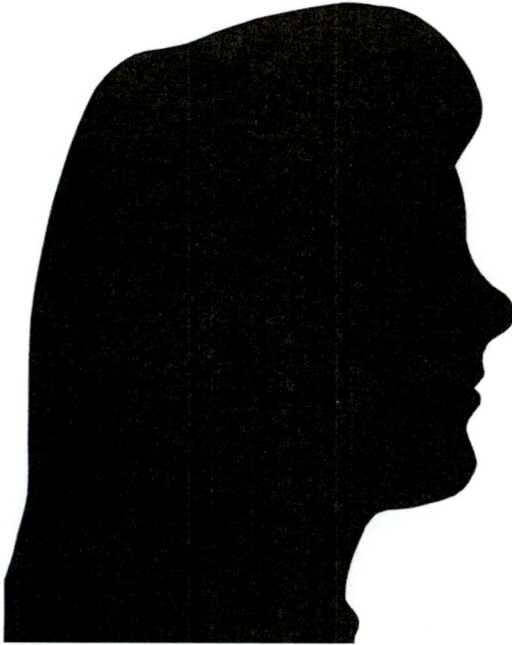

Carole

Love, Dignity, and Alzheimer's
A Journal of
Lessons and Learning

By Gini Cunningham

This book is based on my experiences working
with and learning from loved ones and dear
friends who either have Alzheimer's disease
or who are caregivers for someone with
Alzheimer's or other forms of dementia.

Contact me with your questions or concerns. I
always have an open ear and heart.
gini.cunningham25@gmail.com

Also visit my website for additional
information about Alzheimer's disease.
Together, with knowledge, support, and
research, the mysterious and devastating web
of Alzheimer's disease will be untangled and
solved.
www.lovedignityalzheimers.net

ISBN-10:   1517298016
ISBN-13: 978-1517298012

From the first draft, I have read this book and cried over its pages. The beauty of Gini's writing, used to convey the tragedy and ugliness of Alzheimer's, provides an amazing juxtaposition. I never knew much about Alzheimer's disease until I read "the Carole book" (as we called it) other than the vague bits of information that one picks up from the news, various publications, and conversations with those who announce that a parent has been diagnosed with Alzheimer's. From reading *Love, Dignity, and Alzheimer's – A Journal of Lessons and Learning*, readers will not only gain specific knowledge about this horrendous disease but will also obtain an intimate sense of what happens to families and to individuals who are connected to those with Alzheimer's. It will be impossible for people to read this book and not be changed in their perception and conviction about a disease that is affecting all of us personally, socially, morally, and financially. Before you have finished reading *Love, Dignity, and Alzheimer's*, you will already be telling your friends about it and will be buying copies to give to those you care about. It begs to be discussed and shared. We all need to know more and Gini helps us do that – through her knowledge, her wisdom, and her pain.

~ Meggin McIntosh, Ph.D.

Everyone - doctors, nurses, psychologists, family members, and friends - should read this book, whether it is for Alzheimer's, dementia, a psychiatric disorder or the simple caretaking of an aging loved one with a chronic illness. The book speaks volumes as to how to organize; how to adapt to frustrations; how to manage tyrants; how to deal with embarrassment' and how to find "angels" who show up to help in unexpected places.
The overall arc of the book is a commitment to remembering the human and the heart when all seems haunted by the loss of the person previously known. The book reads like a novel, deeply touches the emotions, and provides a treasure of guidance for families and caretakers alike. The raw courage and struggles of the author provide an inspiration rarely conveyed in self-help resources. I highly recommend this valuable resource!

~ *Linda W. Peterson-St. Pierre PhD*

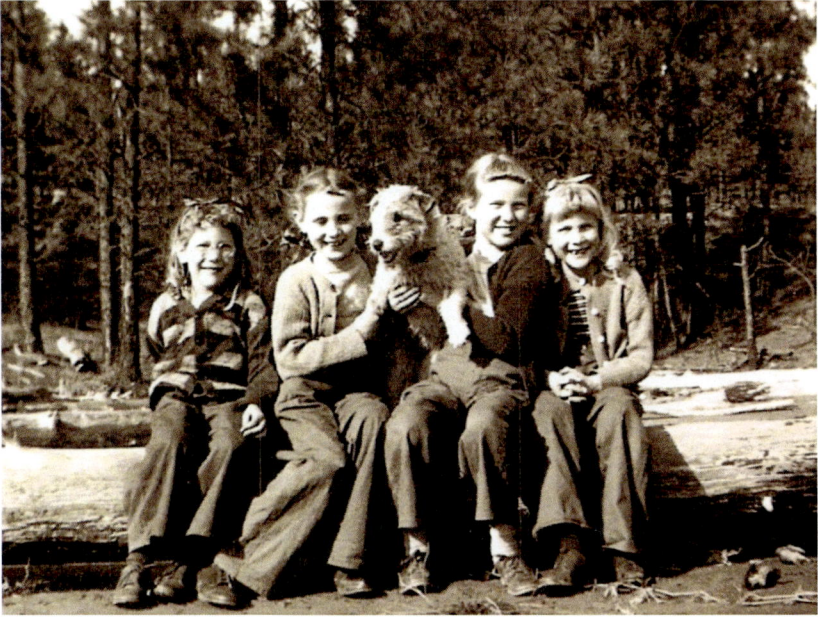

Dedicated to
"The Sisters"
with Love
Jackie, Carole, Marilyn, and Judy with Bumpy
the Dog

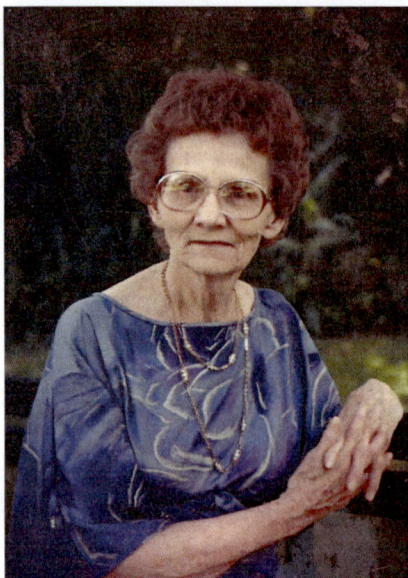

Mama

It is not easy to write about the tragedy of
Alzheimer's disease and yet thee is healing in each
word.
It is hard to begin the word flow…
It is hard to allow it to end…
But much has been gained through
    each reflection,
        each interview,
            each conversation,
                each moment of life.

My dear Mama,
My gentle sister Carole,
My darling friends,
My tender support group members
Every one has provided wisdom and
guidance that I now share with you.

Some of the tales are brimming with humor
because you have to laugh as you navigate this
endless nightmare.

Some of the stories are heartbreaking
because that is the way of Alzheimer's.

As a reader, whether one who suspects dementia, a
caregiver, or just a caring friend, you may want
to scan the Table of Contents to decide what fits
your needs. It has been created in what feels to
me like a sensible order, but this order may differ
from your needs.

You might read read start to finish
or you want to skip and jump and
wind and rewind.

There is no exact pattern.
There is no precise method.

Just know that each word is from my heart, from
my experiences, and all of it is real.

This book is to assist you, to remind you that are not alone, and that there is support.
Writing helps. That is why each chapter has a corresponding section for you to record your thoughts. Writing helps clarify and highlight as it brings buried secrets and emotions to the surface. It is empowering.

With knowledge, research, and desperate desire, Alzheimer's disease will someday be a fading memory.

Ah, the perfect, the ideal definition.
Alzheimer's — a fading Memory.

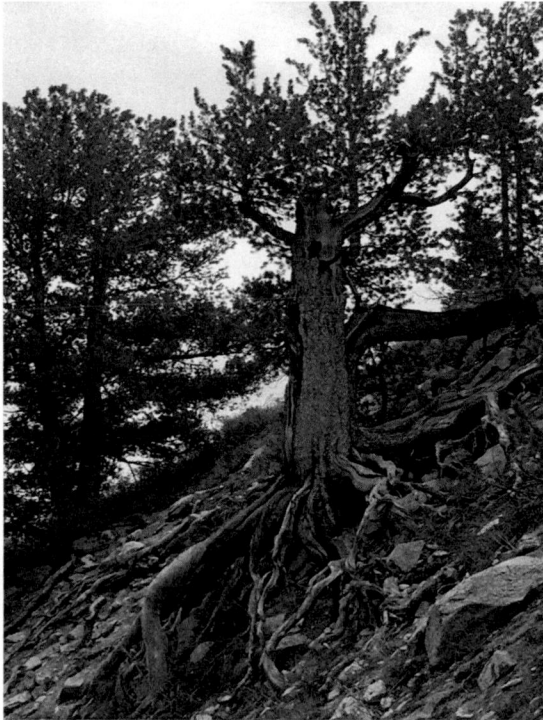

Love, Dignity, and Alzheimer's
A Journal of Lessons and Learning
Table of Contents

Foreword
Love, Dignity, and Alzheimer's
A Journal of Lessons and Learning

As I write this, I am keenly aware that there are thirty-six million people worldwide suffering from dementia. Over five million live in the United States of whom twenty-nine thousand reside in the State of Nevada. In addition, there are at least 200,000 cases of young onset Alzheimer's disease developing in individuals before the age of 65. Young or older onset, slowly over time, Alzheimer's disease robs individuals of their memories, judgment, speech, comprehension, and cognitive abilities that are essential to living daily life.

Alzheimer's disease is the most common form of dementia and while many people believe so, it is not a part of typical aging. The Alzheimer's Association started thirty years ago as a grassroots response to families seeking support, information, and counseling to help them best care for their loved ones with Alzheimer's disease and related dementias. Since then, greater awareness about Alzheimer's disease has occurred, more resources have become available, caregivers have more opportunities to participate in training to enhance their care of the individual with Alzheimer's disease, the condition is diagnosed earlier for more timely interventions, and medications to help slow the progression of the disease have been developed.

But we have light years to go. We need more research and more research dollars to identify the disease earlier and to prevent its progression. We need to create ways for our society to provide respite care for family caregivers so that they will not have to go down the long, difficult path of confusion and pain alone. We still do not have an appropriate long-term care system that is designed to provide help and care affordably—in the home, when possible. Most importantly, we need to learn more about prevention in order to reduce the risk of developing Alzheimer's disease and related dementias.

With public will and political muscle, we are moving forward. There is hope. By creating collaboration between governments, communities, non-governmental organizations, professionals, and most of all, families caring for those with Alzheimer's disease and related dementias, research funding has increased, resources are better designated, and healthcare and community care for persons with Alzheimer's disease and related dementias have been enhanced. We are developing global, national, and state plans to respond to the growing crisis. We will find a solution.

Family caregivers carry the biggest burden of dementia care. At this writing, there are nearly 10 million American family members providing unpaid care for their loved ones with Alzheimer's disease or related dementias. Sixty percent of these family caregivers are women, their average age is forty-eight, and each year they provide $94,000,000,000 worth of unpaid care for loved ones, care which may last for five years or longer. Such care giving has an impact on their health, their employment, their emotional well-being, their income, and their financial security.

The vision of the Alzheimer's Association is to "Imagine a world without Alzheimer's disease." This dream can and will be realized. The Cunninghams and their extended family are planting the seeds and tilling the soil for this vision. These seeds are rooted in the rich soil of love and dignity, which no disease can steal away from those accompanying their loved ones on the journey of Alzheimer's disease. Such families are role models for those of us caring for loved ones. We stand in awe of such families. We honor and thank such families for their courage, insight, and dedication.

Love, Dignity and Alzheimer's – A Journal of Lessons and Learning is one such inspirational story of a family who remembers their loved one with Alzheimer's disease, who embraces the journey of care for her, who reminisces on her life with deep affection. It is the story of those who view life on a much bigger scale than many in our world are able to do. It is a story of everlasting love.

Angie Pratt
Alzheimer's Association
September 2010

Introduction
Making Sense of No Sense - Beginnings and Endings

Carole's Story - Beginnings

More than a decade had elapsed since my sister Jackie's birth when my mother once again heard those stunning words, "You're pregnant." Mama was astounded and my four sisters danced with glee at the thought of a "baby-doll sister", and what did they receive but the independent me! The neighbors, probably in shock with Mama expecting at age forty, gave me the loveliest crib ever. A delightful blue bunny painted on the headboard guarded me as I slept and the softest covers snuggled my little body. I loved it. However, I would later learn that the favored crib came with the label "Six-Year Crib" and for that reason Mama intended that I sleep in it until that age.

There were just two upstairs bedrooms in the house that Daddy had built for us. My oldest sisters, Marilyn and Carole, occupied one. Sisters Judy and Jackie shared the other. During my third year Marilyn moved away to college and Carole gained a bedroom all to herself, but not for long. With a bit of space open, my crib shuffled from my kitchen alcove to my new room with Carole.

When I awakened that first sunny morning, I peeked between the crib bars to Carole who was resting tranquilly across the room. Her soft breathing soothed me as I stared toward her. I felt peaceful and safe with her nearby to protect me. I wiggled to create a few squeaky noises with the crib, just enough to draw her from her sleep. Her left eye popped open over the edge of her pillow and then the other struggled to drag itself awake. These actions led to a smile that glimmered. She quietly pushed back her woolen blanket, dropped her feet onto the cool bedroom floor, and tiptoed toward my bed. Why I did not just climb over the edge of the crib and trundle over to Carole on my own seems odd, but I simply waited for her to lift me into her arms and then hold me close against her warm body. We burrowed deep down into her comfy bed. She soon dozed off again and I lay quiet, serene, and safe.

Sunshine, warmth, tenderness, and safety define my sister Carole. This peaceful, soothing memory of her helps me better cope with the later events of her life, especially those times we lived as she slipped and slid through the depths of Alzheimer's disease. Remembering pleasant scenes broadens my vision and understanding as I work to make sense of no sense.

Carole's Story - Endings

As Carole neared her last breath of life, she again came to me as I peered between bars. This time I leaned against the steely bars of her hospital bed, staring in at the crumpled ball that represented the remnants of my sister. Every bone protruded in skeleton-like clearness. Her eyes sunk into tiny slits that revealed nothing but emptiness. No sparkle, no joy, and no vibrancy emitted from her once happy self. Entrenched in a fetal knot, her tightly bound body consisted of locked bones and emaciated muscles that refused to release. Devilish confusion enveloped her.

Her labored breathing rasped in a jumble of unidentifiable, throaty sounds. I sat helplessly as my sister withdrew from life as Alzheimer's disease dragged her slowly away from my world.

Just after Christmas my husband Lynn and I and our children Stan and Allison had driven from Nevada to California for a brief visit with Carole to deliver our final good-byes. The hospital emergency room doctors had again told my brother-in-law Rich that nothing would reverse the course of the disease and so she now rested at home, waiting for death to swoop her away. Nothing could save her, nothing could restore her life as she and we knew it, nothing could be done except to allow her to leave us within the peace and safety of her family.

Carole's rented bed filled the space where the dining room table had previously stood. The table lay on its side with its worn chairs haphazardly stacked next to it. Caregivers from Visiting Angels remained on duty throughout the day and night to relieve my brother-in-law from full-time care and to make Carole as comfortable as possible. Family assisted as we could. Waiting for death is a dreadful vigil.

Earlier that morning Carole had been lifted into her wheelchair to adjust the weight on her bones and to prevent constant rubbing and more bedsores. Tied into the seat to prevent her from tumbling to the floor, she had been pushed into the glowing sunlight that beamed through the sliding glass doors of the family room. What began as kindness to warm and sooth her over time took on the wretched air of medieval cruelty. Carole sat listlessly, bound mentally and physically in torture from which there was no escape.

Our pats and hugs of reassurance did not seem to reach her. Sensing her exhaustion, we rolled her chair back to the side of her bed and then we encircled her with our arms, lifted her ball-like form from the chair, and gently placed her back onto her soft, white sheets. Carole, however, could not unwind; the tight knot of her body would not unlock. She remained inert, as if frozen, tethered in agony, as we stood by, powerless.

Carole, except for a few labored breaths and wisps of heartbeat, was gone. Erasing this horrifying image, so inhuman and inhumane, has been a struggle. A disease with such a vice-like grip on life is overwhelming. Mercilessly locking one's brain and then stealthily robbing one's body are unimaginable injustices. And when all of this is happening to one you love, your heart is ripped and your emotions stretched almost beyond endurance. I felt angry at the disease, at medicine, at Carole's doctors, at the unfairness of it all. Certainly there must have been an alternative to this tragic end. Why would this happen to someone so kind?

I wanted my Carole back even for just an instant so that she and I could make our good-byes, but to add minutes to this agony was unkind and a selfish. This last glimpse of Carole, this frightful picture, possessed me. Understanding eluded me for months as I worked to eliminate this nightmare view and return to a joyful memory of Carole. I was helpless to reverse Carole's life ending as I struggled to grant her peace to go.

My Story

Memories of Carole and those of my mother who also died of Alzheimer's disease plus the other individuals with Alzheimer's and their caregivers are shared in this book to help you better understand the possible symptoms, progressions, emotions, and the ominous reality of this terrible disease. My connections to Alzheimer's disease have been close-up and personal; the words I share with you come from my heart, my personal experiences and those of others who have been willing to share with me, plus there are so many lessons that I have learned along the way. I have read and researched many angles and aspects of Alzheimer's disease to try to better understand it and to find ways to reassure others that there is hope.

The precise pattern of Alzheimer's progression is allusive, but there are many manifestations of the disease that are common to most individuals who have it. Fortunately the symptoms do not always lead to Alzheimer's disease, but they may lead to diagnosis of the probability of the disease and rule out other causes of change or mental decline.

Alzheimer's shares symptoms with many other dementias. Only a thorough examination by a neurologist, one specifically trained in the diagnosis and treatment options of Alzheimer's and other dementias can provide you and your loved one with the valuable information needed to support you as you face the possibilities of this disease.

My mom had about four years of sinking into Alzheimer's disease until her death at seventy-nine years. I could rationalize her passing to a degree because of her age; she had lived a rich, long life and she had accomplished much. Carole's first symptoms of the disease that only became truly visible in hindsight began in her early fifties and struck full-force by her sixtieth birthday. Seven more years of the disease engulfed her until death at the age of sixty-seven. It is bewildering how the disease strikes and how it carries out its death sentence.

Volunteering as facilitator for my local Alzheimer's Support Group has taught me even more about this disease and has provided me with stories and perspectives of our members. The Winnemucca Alzheimer's Support Group, the Northern Nevada Alzheimer's Association, The Alzheimer's Day Care Facility in San Jose, and the national Alzheimer's Association have enriched my knowledge and understanding. This knowledge echoes throughout *Love, Dignity, and Alzheimer's - A Journal of Lessons and Learning* and repeats the message of the love and dignity that are so critical to the well being of the loved one with the disease and the caregivers who confront this fierce monster.

Insight and Understanding

From Carole and Mama I gained insight and understanding. From research and writing hope has been revived and I have reclaimed fragments of wholeness. The pain has lessened but it still exists in my heart. I've drawn on many sources to create this book of love, lessons, and learning. Stories and experiences are shared with the belief that this knowledge can help you, as a caregiver, a family member, or someone with Alzheimer's or other dementia. Each reader's lens will view aspects of this disease differently; knowledge will arrive from different angles with different perceptions and perspectives; connectedness and understanding will grow as certain symptoms or scenarios directly target you and other points (fortunately) bounce away. May the stories and information support you through the Alzheimer's journey as you learn to make sense of no sense.

Stories from my family and me use our given names; the names in the stories from my support group have been changed to maintain their privacy. So many individuals have been integral in the recapturing of memories and placing them into print for readers everywhere. I know that many of these will touch you, change your thinking, and assure you that you are not alone.

Bars to hold us in as in safe little cribs; bars to keep us out as in steely hospital beds; memories tied to my childhood crib and then to Carole's deathbed. How uniquely circular and well planned is the story of life.

After Carole was gone, I struggled to superimpose the picture of my beautiful, delicate sister on top of the nightmare of her dying. Alzheimer's disease produces prolonged pain and leaves a frightening image as residue. Learning to refocus and re-envision have brought me peace and wisdom.

While it is never easy to lose someone close to our hearts, Alzheimer's extends the ache as a loved one melts into oblivion. But even at the end, Carole remained with me. Though seemingly unresponsive, caught in sticky bonds of disconnection, she "knew" me when and how she could. I did not understand her mumbled words or strange gestures; sense had long since vanished. But I truly believe even though she could not recall my name or possibly even recognize me, she felt the love and the wish for dignity that I offered her.

Some will say that someone with Alzheimer's is completely lost and that no connection with the outside world exists; my experiences tell me that that is not true. The love may be ensnared but it lives; dignity resides.

A single blessing of Alzheimer's, although blessing is an anomalous term when associated with this disease, is that as the illness progresses, the person with Alzheimer's disease appears to be less and less aware of the stripping away of every shred of humanity and independence. While loved ones watch in horror as the disease intensifies its grip, glimmers of deep understanding become fainter for the one with dementia. I hope and pray this is true because I cannot imagine the torture of realizing the persistent devastation of one's mental capacity while being entirely powerless to reverse it. When awareness does arise in the victim, it appears to last but a millisecond so that the total catastrophic nature of Alzheimer's is not fully comprehended. This conjecture of "unawareness" lessens the anguish of those of us who are forced to stand by helplessly, hoping for better days while preparing for worse. Those on the outside view the destruction, but the victim seems to sense it only in brief wisps of lucidity.

Reviving Hope

Carole clung to life with unfeasible power. But in hindsight, she preferred to do things in her own way and so she waited until New Year's Day to leave this world and enter her next. I believe that somehow, even in the throes of this wicked departure, she was protecting her husband Rich. In this case she wanted him to have an income tax deduction for the ensuing year. It sounds crazy, even outlandish and almost silly, I know, but she would have been searching for a way to help Rich as he learned to stand without her.

You may think that this shift from dying to income tax is too sudden, almost too humorous or callous, but it imitates the way of Alzheimer's: in then out, up then down, cognizant then unaware, patterned then confused. Carole had been a strong, effervescent being; her Alzheimer's shell only represented the end of her life. With Alzheimer's and other dementias it is sometimes easy to "forget" the unique individual who dwells within. But even in the worst of times, even with her inability to reveal her precise thoughts and desires, she was with us in her own special way.

Hope is essential when traveling along the Alzheimer's road. Hope allows for bits of light and later leads to eventual healing and recovery from dying and death. Hope requires patience, forgiveness of the victim as well as of oneself, and it can take many months and years to acquire. Hope brings acceptance that also brings renewal and peace. Some people never quite regain their faith in anything of value. They struggle until their own death with anger and anguish and little or no rebirth of hope for the future. It is important to know that the loved one swathed in dementia, the loved one who has passed away, wants those who remain to mend and live. Recognizing the innocence of the victim of this horrendous disease and then working to recall and revive the happiness of the past carry healing, health, and hope as survivors find ways to endure and revive from this dark disease.

Becoming Whole

Regaining a healthy outlook and clear focus requires many things including:

- **Time:** Days, weeks, months, years; in time there can be joy again; recovery time varies and it may be inconsistent from day to day, week to week, or throughout life.
- **Patience:** Within yourself, for the loved one with the disease, and with and from others; we all face dying and death in our own ways and recovering from both is individual and unique.
- **Understanding:** Alzheimer's disease is a long, torturous, one-way descent; there are no simple, easy steps.
- **Forgiveness:** In a variety of forms forgiveness encompasses forgiving yourself, your loved one, how others may have acted or reacted, the unexplainable behaviors and events that have transpired, and finally the disease itself.
- **Belief:** In the goodness of life and of those we love; Alzheimer's is a slow, treacherous disease but you will learn to appreciate every bright moment that

19

arises and the multitude of lessons that will be learned. You will be changed in many ways.

- **Acceptance: Life can go on; renewal and revival are possible. There is hope.**

Each chapter of *Love, Dignity, and Alzheimer's – A Journal of Lessons and Learning* is designed to assist you through the toughest of times. The stories are factual, the people with Alzheimer's and their caregivers are real, and the family survivors are brave as they share their experiences and their growth in knowledge plus reveal their wisdom and desire to help others. Those with the disease and caregivers often feel so isolated but there are people and abundant resources to provide information and support. As you read on you will learn many of these.

Renewal Resources

Each chapter includes stories of my experiences with people with Alzheimer's and families affected by Alzheimer's disease. There are subsections labeled: "Insight and Understanding", "Reviving Hope", "Becoming Whole", and "Renewal Resources". Each section is designed to enhance your knowledge of Alzheimer's disease, to share possible stages of the disease and emotions that may accompany you on this journey, and advice and lessons learned by me and by others with whom I work that may alleviate or circumvent potential problems for you.

All words are from my heart. Neither a trained medical professional nor an expert in the field, experience uniquely qualifies me to share lessons learned as a caregiver for and surviving witness of loved ones with Alzheimer's disease. There are many books, articles, and websites with information on the disease. Research and read those that support your struggle and bring you help.

To guide you as you face the Alzheimer's dilemma and to help you regain happiness and clear vision, activities for each chapter have been included in **APPENDIX I**. The pain and confusion you have endured can be transformed into lessons and learning through reflection and writing. Refer to Memory Activity Introduction under *Healing: Reflection and Writing Activities* (page 130) to supplement the information in the Introduction of *Love, Dignity, and Alzheimer's*. Reflection and writing are tools that have helped me recapture a sense of purpose and they are tools that can support you as well.

Facts and Figures

- Of the top 10 killers, Alzheimer's ranks #6. It is the only one that cannot be prevented, cured, or even slowed

- Nearly 1 in every 5 Medicare dollar is spent on people with Alzheimer's disease.

- Less than 45% of individuals who have Alzheimer's disease are told so by their physicians.

- Only 33% of Americans diagnosed with Alzheimer's are aware that they have it.

- In 2013 over 84,000 Americans died *from* Alzheimer's disease.

- In 2015 over 700,000 Americans will die *with* Alzheimer's disease, meaning the death certificate will indicate something different even thought AD was the underlying cause.

- 60% of Caregivers of individuals with Alzheimer's and other dementias report high emotional stress.

- 40% of Caregivers of individuals with Alzheimer's and other dementias report depression.

- Today 5.6-5.8 million Americans are living with Alzheimer's disease.

- Nearly 2/3 of those with Alzheimer's disease are women.

- Someone in the United States develops Alzheimer's disease every 67 seconds.

- Changes in the brain are associated with Alzheimer's disease. As plaques and tangles develop, neurons are unable to fire between synapses. As synapses fail, the number of synapses declines and neurons eventually die.

- Genetic mutations, an abnormal change in the sequence of chemical pairs, causes memory failure and Alzheimer's disease

Chapter 1
Initial Symptoms
Actions and Reactions

Jodi's Story – my aunt and Alzheimer's

Alzheimer's is such a mean disease. I recall speaking with my aunt when she discovered that she was in its early stages. She and my uncle were traveling home from a vacation and they stopped by our home. She shared with me the numerous medications that she was taking and her hope that they would slow down the progress of this insidious disease. I remember feeling helpless as to what to say to her. I just gave her a hug and told her that everything was going to be okay. As I look back on it now, I wish that I had asked her, "How can I help?" Although her thinking at the time was a bit muddled, she was still my sweet aunt.

As her disease progressed, my aunt slipped further away … her eyes became more and more unfocused and she seemed more and more removed. However, true to her nature, her love of children and animals remained. Alzheimer's is terrible disease to witness as you watch someone you love melt into its grasp. Near the end of her life I saw anger come through in my sweet-natured aunt. My feeling was that this was due to frustration of losing a sense of control. How can something so cruel besiege someone so dear?

Actions and Reactions

It is difficult to imagine how a victim endures the nagging suspicion of the presence of a disease like Alzheimer's. It is one thing to misplace an income tax form and later discover it peeking out of the garbage where it has been stuffed with a pile of other seemingly worthless documentation. It is quite another to have this "forgetfulness" return again and again. Lost papers, keys, shoes, sense of directions, recognition of formerly familiar faces… No book, no research, no doctor's advice can adequately prepare a loved one with Alzheimer's disease for this terrifying knell nor can they prepare the caregiver and family. Current medications treat symptoms of the disease, but they do not prevent or cure this frightening culprit.

As my mother began to forget she protected herself by placing the daily newspaper on her table, circling the date, and attaching notes for meetings and other scheduled events to prod her memory and keep her on track (and she fooled her daughters into inaction). Her reminders served her well as she worked to maintain a fairly independent life, and allowed me to deny repeatedly that anything was wrong with her other than a touch of poor memory. Later when my sister Carole began to show signs of the disease, I should have immediately recognized the warning symptoms that she displayed. With Carole, I was more aware of her forgetting because I had seen it so recently with Mama, but I was also very adept at denying the disease because I knew that only a tragic outcome existed. My sister had always been a little scatter-brained and so forgetting seemed normal; plus she was so young, in her early fifties, there just couldn't be anything seriously wrong.

Regardless of the evidence, denial often helps one control extraordinary stress and anxiety. Repeated denial can feel like the truth; it can be comforting until one is finally ready to face the clamoring wake-up call. I eventually had to admit that repeatedly forgetting dates, purses, appointments, directions, and telephone numbers was beyond normal. As the veil of denial disintegrated I was forced to confront the possibility that Alzheimer's disease had invaded my mom and later my sister. It is a process that many of the caregivers with whom I have worked have reiterated. Denial provides distance, a sense of safety, and possibilities of hope; admitting the truth is not easy. "Forgetting" may or may not signal Alzheimer's disease and so it is essential that you rule things out like a UTI infection or poor medication combination as you educate yourself on the many forms of dementia, one of which is Alzheimer's disease.

Insight and Understanding

Even when a diagnosis is given, Alzheimer's is a strange enemy. Sometimes it is obviously present and caregivers as well as the one diagnosed knows and recognizes that something is just not right. It may begin with questions like: "Where are my keys?" "Which street do I turn on?"

"Who left the stove on?" Questions once in a while are no problem, right? When questions recur with recurring arguments and vengeance, a problem definitely is present. As Alzheimer's seeps into one's brain, the lapses of memory expand. "Where are my keys?" becomes a daily routine and then suspicion enters. You diligently search for the keys and when you, as caregiver, locate them on the table (in plain view) and try to hand them over you are greeted with, "Why do you have my keys? Why did you hide them? Never touch them again!"

Anger mounts as the ridiculousness of the accusation intensifies. No apologizes or explanations suffice, and if you become angry in what feels like justifiable return, problems only escalate. Arguing with a person who is confused with dementia is not a winnable situation. Never.

Then suddenly the key accusation is dropped and life returns to normal. The lost keys are temporarily found, the anger dissipates, and eventually the entire trauma of the moment vanishes from memory. If you bring up, "Remember the last time..." a blank stare of disbelief may appear which may then be replaced by a return to anger if you pursue the conversation. This lag in memory may also be laced with fear for the victim, especially if he has witnessed this voracious disease in others. A wink of suspicion of cognitive deterioration can be devastating. Imagine visualizing it within yourself.

Mama hid her knowledge of the disease until it was hurtled into her face. She had been active in a group called Century Club, a philanthropic organization. She had held several offices, attended regularly, and donated generously. For the fall gathering she had been assigned the responsibility of refreshments. As an early morning meeting was scheduled, she decided on donuts as snacks. She called Mildred to bring a dozen; then she called Maxine; then Angela, Patricia, Clara, Zelda, and ... She forgot that she had called these friends, and so she called more. To be sure that there were enough, she also brought three dozen extra. Donuts covered the tables, the chairs, and filled the room. Mama was embarrassed at her error but she smiled nevertheless. After all, it was a minor error, a silly mistake. Helga, the president, however, was not so inclined. She scathingly berated Mama, in private before the meeting, in front of others during the meeting, and again at its end. She followed Mama out into the parking lot, harangued her once more, and left her in tears. Mama dropped out of the organization, and in fact she quit every outside club to which she had belonged after this incident.

As her daughter I wondered why she had stopped the clubs that she had enjoyed so much as I encouraged her to maintain her active lifestyle. Only months later did she reveal the dreadful, insensitive attack. Why would she ever want to attend anything ever again? And I was left with uncertainty and worry. What was happening to my Mama?

By the time Alzheimer's disease was fully evident Carole was mired in its depths and she appeared helpless to fight it other than in sporadic outbursts as she struggled unsuccessfully to beat it away. Her anger was out of character and I believe her outbursts exemplified her frustration with this futile fight as she struck out in the only conceivable way she could.

TW's Story — Carole's Fury

We were enjoying a pleasant afternoon at our cabin. I was out on the dock reading when suddenly Aunt Carole attacked. For hours she had been tromping up and down the beach muttering, crossing the little bridge to the dock, pausing, muttering, pivoting, and then re-tromping the beach. Occasionally her words were clear, "Don't you do that; don't you ever do that." This frustrated appeal had been used often during that vacation and I always just nodded and smiled, "OK, Aunt Carole. I won't do it again," even though the "that" was incomprehensible to me.

On this particular march down the dock Carole stopped, glared, shouted her epitaph, and then she wadded her fist and conked me on the head. She wheeled in anger, shuffled off the dock and down the beach. My gentle aunt had transformed into viciousness. A few minutes later, Carole returned with renewed fury. As I readied for her onslaught as her fist shadowed my head, she stopped in midair, uncoiled her hand, and then gently patted my head. "I'm sorry, I'm so sorry," came from the depths of her being. Clear, recognizable words strung together in meaning choked out, more words than she had uttered in sequence for months. Then she turned and renewed her wandering trudge, forgetting the scene in an instant.

As time goes by essential life skills suddenly go astray as gaps in abilities, correct word choice and problems with sequencing or following directions appear, and formerly natural skills disappear. *As time goes by* and *suddenly* seem to contradict each other but they correspond well to a disease that manifests itself in its sly manner: slowly, tick by tick, relentlessly, and then unexpectedly the explicable becomes inexplicable. And then with equal suddenness the inexplicable is explained.

When the severity of the crisis becomes impossible to deny, even though denial feels the safest and best way to continue living, truth materializes. Re-entering denial on occasion because of its recognizable safety is common, just as admitting the existence of the disease feels as if hope has been dashed. However, admitting the possibility of Alzheimer's disease clears the way for reality and possible interventions and medications.

Pinpointing the precise time for help is tricky; in one instant, skills have vanished and the known world melts; then back the memories and abilities flood. "I do not know how to tie my shoes" puzzlement spreads across a loved one's face and then abruptly she sits down and ties them. Relief flows in because a skill has returned and then it is sidetracked by the troubling question, "Who are you?" This back and forth confusion is exhausting and scary, but it is often the nudge needed to admit that a problem exists.

As lucid moments become fewer and the opportunity to retreat from the fear of Alzheimer's disappears, families tackle the facts of the disease; accepting the need for support, advice, and help is important. "Just a memory lapse..." carries dwindling relief. The comfort previously found in believing that the forgetfulness worry is unfounded and just a temporary bump for today, is drowned when repeated forgetting becomes unending, potentially dangerous, and the security of denial becomes insecure.

Alzheimer's is a continuous descent with plateaus along the way. These leveling off periods provide the opportunity to sort of "catch up" and regroup for the next physical or mental loss.

Reviving Hope

Maybe Alzheimer's comes as it does, in small doses and tiny steps, to warn the victim and the family of what lies ahead. Maybe that is a snippet of kindness that comes with this disease. While I take little solace in this, it is somewhat helpful to think that it may provide a warning sign for me and my own possibility of the disease or for others who are caring for someone who appears to have dementia. Perhaps the slow entry process allows time to prepare. Maybe in the tangle these flashes of hope, these splashes of lucidity, life continues in a fashion that feels complete and free from anguish for a little longer.

Loved ones with Alzheimer's are blameless individuals upon whom this disease has set aim. They are often misunderstood because their actions and reactions are out of the norm. As bystanders, if the loved one is Dad or Grandma, we have pleasant memories to fall back on, connections of happiness and personal value to support the horror of the disease. To outsiders, however, those with Alzheimer's may appear strange and creepy. With hair askew, hygiene amiss, and inhibition run rampant, those with no relationship to your loved one may laugh, gawk, or tremble with outrage. Most often people with Alzheimer's, especially as the disease progresses, do not recognize this vicious perception, but to family members the pain can be unbearable. There is little positive reaction possible when others deride and ridicule. Bravery to stand tall and forgive the uninformed is a characteristic that will help you.

Sadly, too, some family members may be too terrified of the symptoms of the disease to remember that Grandpa still resides within. Adult children may be afraid to visit; aunts and uncles may act as if the disease is contagious. Fortunately most young children simply love. They have the magical ability to see beyond the cruel manifestations of the disease to the individual wrapped inside. This is not true during times of violence, as some people with Alzheimer's have unreasonable and inexplicable lashing out occasions that wound. But children are forgiving and are able to look forward to a next visit when Great Grandma will be calm and loving once again.

Pets are also forgiving of the victim and often become very protective. A gentle dog or cat offers enormous comfort to one with Alzheimer's disease as a companion and non-judgmental friend. Children and pets perceive innocence.

Renewal Resources

There are many facts to learn about the initial stages of Alzheimer's disease. First know and recognize the 10 potential symptoms. As you read through the list remember that these *may* be signs, but forgetfulness can come from many other quarters besides dementia and Alzheimer's disease. Urinary tract infections, depression, stress, nutritional imbalance, strokes, and more can cause dementia-like characteristics. And while Alzheimer's is a slow, progressive, degenerative disease, it is just one form of dementia; not all dementias are Alzheimer's. A thorough examination by the family physician rules out some possible causes for memory and behavior changes; a complete examination by a qualified neurologist provides more insight, information, and correct diagnosis and treatment plan.

Initial Symptoms

1. **Memory Loss**
   Forgetting recently learned information is one of the common signs of Alzheimer's. A person forgets more often and is unable to recall information later.

2. **Difficulty performing familiar tasks.**
   People with Alzheimer's often find it hard or impossible to plan everyday tasks. They may forget how to follow directions, play a game, or make a phone call.

3. **Problems with language.**
   People with Alzheimer's disease often forget simple words or substitute unusual words, making their speech or writing hard to understand. They may be unable to find their toothbrush, for example, and instead ask for "that thing with stubs for my mouth clean."

4. **Orientation to time and place**
   People with Alzheimer's may become lost in their own neighborhood, forget how they arrived

somewhere, and be unable to return home after a trip to the store or a friend's home.

5. **Poor or decreased judgment**
   People with Alzheimer's may dress in appropriately for the weather. They may have trouble with money decisions – banking, giving money away, and forgetting to pay bills...

6. **Trouble with abstract reasoning**
   Someone with Alzheimer's may have unusual difficulties completing complex mental tasks like forgetting what numbers represent and their purpose in an equation.

7. **Misplacing things**
   A person with Alzheimer's may put things in unusual places like a ring in a heater vent or the phone in the freezer.

8. **Changes in mood or behavior**
   Someone with Alzheimer's may display sudden mood swings – from calm to agitated to angry – for no apparent reason.

9. **Changes in personality**
   People with Alzheimer's may become extremely suspicious, confused, fearful, or dependent.

10. **Loss of initiative**
    A person with Alzheimer's may become very passive, sitting in front of the television for hours, sleeping more than usual, or not wanting to participate in previously enjoyable activities.
    (Modified from the Alzheimer's Association website)

While each of these is a potential indicator of Alzheimer's disease your doctor and neurologist and your careful observations and journaling are the best sources for diagnosis and intervention.

Refer to **Memory Activity #1** (page 133) in **APPENDIX I** *Healing: Reflection and Writing Activities* to support the information in this chapter, "Initial Symptoms: Actions and Reactions." Reflection and writing are tools that have clarified many aspects and events of Alzheimer's disease for me. They have the potential to help you dig deeply as you work to understand some of the symptoms and behaviors of Alzheimer's disease.

The appearance of the disease may be recognizable and then you will think that the signs have faded and almost disappeared, leaving you with just a suspicion of a problem. Then they may reappear in a slightly different form. The appearance and progression of the disease are as certain as they are uncertain.

But there is understanding and there is hope for remaining connected and attuned to the needs and desires of the Alzheimer's victim. Love, respect, and dignity are powerful instruments of compassion for enduring difficult times.

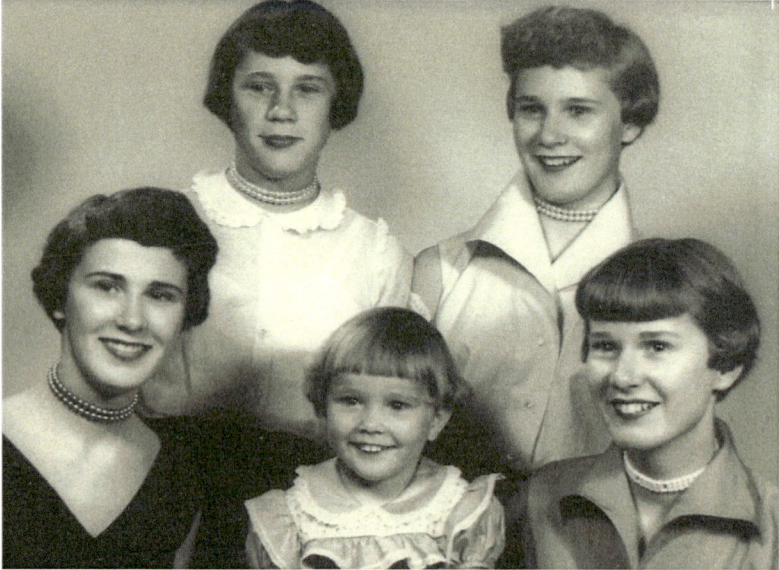
The 5 of Us: Carole, Jackie, Gini, Judy, Marilyn

Notes and Reminders:

Chapter 2
Admitting a Problem
Receiving a Diagnosis
Traveling the Emotional Gambit

Gwen's Story – My first Support Group meeting
Walking into the Quiet Room of our local hospital I was immediately struck by a mix of wild, almost uncontrollable emotions. I had known about the local Alzheimer's Support Group, I had received emails and booklets from the group facilitator, I had chatted with a longtime friend. But leaving denial and admitting I needed help was not easy. In fact I had stalled for weeks until the letter arrived with the diagnosis from the doctor: dementia; potential Alzheimer's.

I picked up a brochure that sat on the table and as I read tears rolled. My husband was just 61, how could this be happening to him? To us? Little tics from his head and shoulder as he drove the work bus led a co-worker to report him to a supervisor. Testing with the company doctor with trivial questions like "Who is the governor" (he gave our previous governor instead of the present one) sealed his fate: frontal-temporal dementia. The furlough papers arrived labeled "Short-term Disability" and its meaning resonated doom, frustration, and worry.

Another doctor, a neurologist, nodded affirmation of the diagnosis. "Seek guardianship," he announced to me as he handed me a prescription. As our questions poured out, he turned and left the room, leaving our echoing voices reverberating in our ears. Yes, my husband was having trouble with naming items, and yes, there had been temporary twitches on his right side, but nothing had indicated he should be placed on irreversible disability with job termination waiting. No sign had been severe enough to warn us that his job would be gone, a job he had faithfully held for 36 years. Nothing had prepared us for an empty diagnosis, a quick prescription, and a void of dignity. No one should ever be treated like this.

Admitting a Problem

Denying the existence of a disease is common; it can even be helpful in protecting your loved one as you sort through medical and financial decisions and research possible solutions to health issues. Admitting a need for help is an enormous step to take, and it should be a step that produces positive results. The doctors in Gwen's case behaved abysmally. Imagine the struggle in recognizing that maybe recent memory lapses and tics are a threat to healthy functioning and then finding the courage to admit that something is not right followed by seeking medical advice. Imagine a doctor who reads "dementia" into not knowing the governor of your state. Imagine a second doctor whose advice is medication and legal restrictions but no discussion about possible help and intervention. No one should be treated with the lack of dignity that Gwen and her husband received.

Receiving a Diagnosis

In 1986 (about four years before her death from Alzheimer's) Mama still lived independently. Meals-on-Wheels delivered hot lunches each day and the wonderful driver made my mom her last delivery so that she could chat, re-warm the food if needed, and provide Mama's daughters who lived far away with extra peace of mind. In the spring Mama visited her physician who requested further testing. He recognized forgetfulness that was troubling so off we went for an "expert" opinion and MRI. The expert poked, prodded, and tapped my mom. He began to deliver his dreadful diagnosis when he decided that Mama was too dim to understand. He turned toward my sister Judy and me and pronounced, "Alzheimer's, dementia. Put her in a home." He reached for the door handle, yanked it open, and left.

We glanced at Mama as tears rimmed her eyes. "No one is supposed to live forever anyway," she told us. She had understood every word the doctor had said; only her difficulty with hearing had prevented a speedy response and thus the doctor had judged her incapable of understanding. In retrospect I wonder how much her deafness played into his dementia decision. Why would a trained physician behave with such insensitivity?

Later that week Judy took Mama to the ordered MRI. Judy watched as the attendants shoved our mother into the steely capsule. She listened as machines vibrated to life. She stared as Mama's feet trembled. When the scan was done and Mama was rolled out into the lighted room, tears dripped from her frightened eyes. Judy quietly patted her and said, "No more. No more tests, Mama." Mama sighed with relief. Mama did have Alzheimer's disease, she did forget many things, but she remained a person.

That summer Mama moved from her home in Nampa. Wheels and hitch were reattached to her mobile home and in a day her residence traveled 70 miles down the road, just a few miles from Judy's home. She lived alone for several months but forgetting to turn off burners and turn up furnaces helped us make the decision to transfer her to assisted living. When the assisted living home suddenly closed, Judy hired fulltime caregivers so that Mama could return home. Thanks to Judy's decision to end useless testing, a local doctor's goodness, and tender caregivers, love and dignity surrounded Mama as her life drew to a close.

Insight and Understanding

Admitting that there is cognitive decline and a decrease in independent functioning is painful and should not be aggravated by inept and uncaring medical personnel. There are trained specialists who understand aging and dementia. Make certain that you and your loved one receive a diagnosis from a doctor who cares about quality of living life, one who understands dementia and the decline of mental ability, one knowledgeable about the process of aging, and one who will listen to the questions and concerns of loved one and caregiver.

Traveling through denial, that safe and comfortable state, and then recognizing and admitting that a problem is not going away lead to possible intervention and help. Tender emotions may unleash other sentiments as well. Sometimes these come on calmly and gradually; at other times they ignite with explosive intensity. They may be mixed in an uncontrollable tumble, they may be vague and wavering, or there may be many combinations. I can now look back and identify the denial, admitting, anger, blame, helplessness, guilt, regret, forgiveness, and eventual acceptance of what was happening to my mom and to Carole but in the midst of it all, I was lost. No feeling entered in a prescribed manner and then exited on cue. There was no circle of emotions that marched forward in a step-by-step, clear-cut sequence. My feelings vacillated back and forth, up and down, around and around but each was tied to love hemmed in by the utter hopelessness of not being able to protect my Mama or sister.

Although you often hear death and dying in that order, doesn't the death come last, and the dying simply lead up to it? Perhaps with Alzheimer's disease, death belongs to the one who is suffering, but dying belongs to each family member who stands by impotently as the disease wrings away the life of its victim. Alzheimer's dying is one of emotional upheaval that lasts for years. Is sudden death preferable? No. Death in my mind is always incomprehensible in its finality. But the slow, protracted Alzheimer's death injures again and again and again. Just when you believe that your loved one has reached a plateau, that the next months will be level with little decline, a new loss arises (refer to Chapter 3 Circuits that Are Not Circuitous for more details on loss of abilities).

In sudden death grief attacks in a flash, with feelings shattered as disbelief and horror set in. With Alzheimer's grief is a constant companion. First, it begins almost imperceptibly and catches one off guard as skills, mental functions, and vitality slip away from someone who is otherwise seemingly healthy. The change is often so minute that it is easily overlooked. Alzheimer's is a slow progression, typically 2-20- years and so dying by degrees typifies its path.

In younger on-set Alzheimer's the victim may endure twenty years of decline. Time passes as the victim gradually loses abilities: oral and written communication, understanding of conversations, ambulation, attending to daily routines and hygiene, and eventually eating, swallowing, and breathing.

Alzheimer's strikes caregivers as well. Loving spouses rearrange plans for retirement, travel, and exploration as unending caregiving enters. Children, especially daughters, become caregivers, too, sometimes later in life after their own children are grown, and at other times adult children raise their own young ones as they care for their parents or grandparents.

"Stages of Grief" is a familiar reference and description for the emotions of loss. It encompasses the combination of feelings that accompany individuals when separation, tragedy, or death arises. Navigating grief is not lock-step. Having lived grief I can identify with floods of emotions that hit then recede and then return in a new form. If grief were patterned, those who hurt would simply march along until suddenly the pain vanished and acceptance flooded in.

I do not see grief as a process either. Process denotes another sequential procedure that ends with precision and healing. Grief is rarely if ever precise and healing is complex. Anger, blame, helplessness, and more comprise the kaleidoscope of grieving. It is complicated and uniquely individual. Often grief can be understood after time or from a distance but it is nearly impossible to understand it when you are in its midst.

I have chosen the title "Enduring Grief" as this depicts Alzheimer's slow, painful advancement, the hours, days, weeks, months, and years that pass as you travel from the initial suspicion to the ultimate loss of a loved one. Survivors witness as a formerly capable being departs a productive life. While hundreds of sentiments exist, I have narrowed the focus to nine, the nine that hit the hardest and the most frequently when one faces the tears (droplets from the eye) and tears (rips in the heart) of an Alzheimer's death. These emotions are not cyclical, they do not come in any specific order, and every individual does not feel them totally or in the same way. We each grieve on our own terms and differences abound in our actions and reactions.

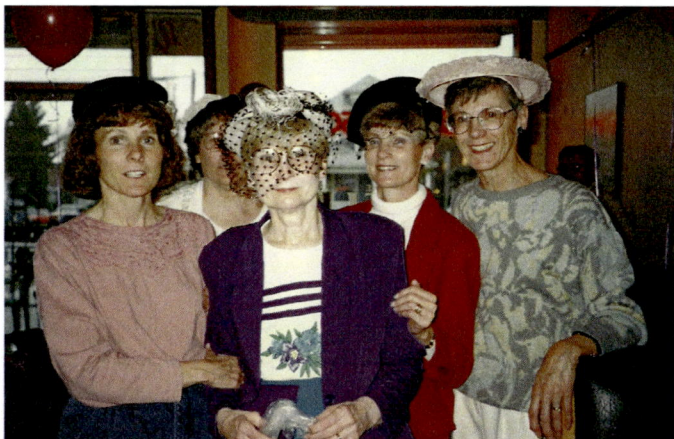

Donning Our Grandmother Peggy's Hats

Traveling the Emotional Gambit

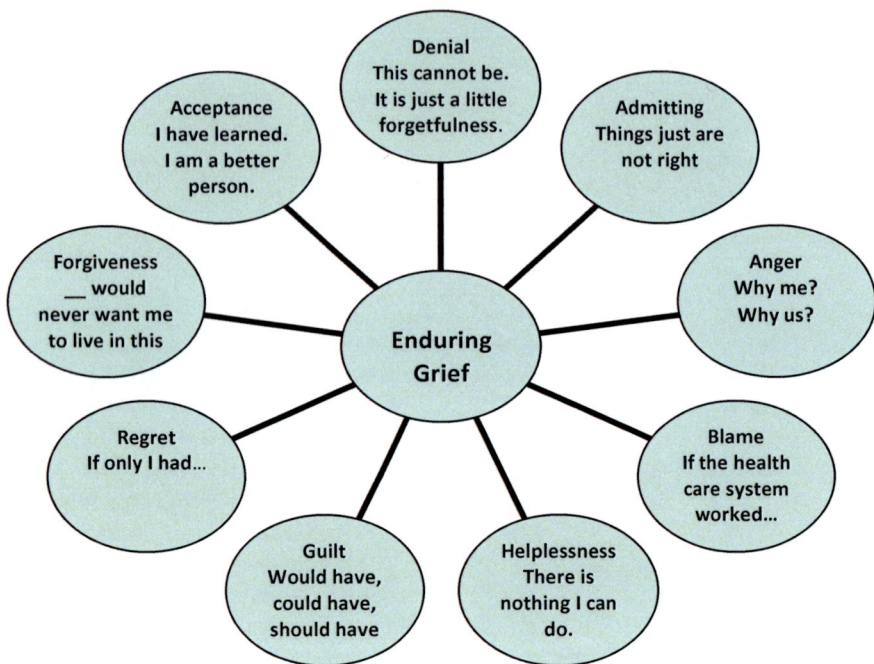

Denial
This cannot be.
It is just a little
forgetfulness.

Acceptance
I have learned.
I am a better
person.

Admitting
Things just are
not right

Forgiveness
__ would
never want me
to live in this

Anger
Why me?
Why us?

**Enduring
Grief**

Regret
If only I had…

Blame
If the health
care system
worked…

Guilt
Would have,
could have,
should have

Helplessness
There is
nothing I can
do.

While enduring grief, feelings enter and leave, return and then vanish, transform, and re-enter. They may stay for a time, and then melt away; they may linger or perhaps move to obscurity. All of these feeling are possible elements of grief and finding a way through them is part of healing from overwhelming loss. You may experience some of these; you may experience them all. They are equally as predictable as they are unpredictable. In working with many people of many ages, variation and complexity of grief are "normal" and through living them and attempting to understand them, there can be acceptance and forgiveness. But reaching that level takes time.

Just as you will experience a range of feelings, so will those that you love: family members, friends, as well as the individual with Alzheimer's who dies a little bit each day. Some may deny the existence of a problem right up to the end; others long for a quick diagnosis and fast movement into assisted living or a long-term care facility. Some might be angry while others seek blame. Alzheimer's disease is nearly impossible to make sense of and the actions surrounding it and reactions toward it are widely scattered. Patience and understanding are two attributes that support you during this journey of loss: patience and understanding for the victim, for yourself, and for everyone else who touches your life.

Reviving Hope
Grief strangles emotional well-being; only time, support from others, and personal effort lead to the containment and management of grief. This in turn leads to individual healing and hopefully family healing. The following definitions for the nine sentiments felt while Enduring Grief reflect my own emotional struggle with Alzheimer's disease. Emotions are personal in intensity and meaning, but this guide offers insight that may help you.

- **Denial** – Denial is the refusal to admit or even consider that there is a problem, a worry, and a concern. Ah, there is bliss and safety in pegging odd moments onto forgetfulness! Denial is safe, secure, and offers protection from reality. Some may never emerge from this stage; others readily accept a diagnosis and medical evidence and prepare to move forward.

- **Admitting** – A frequent first step in moving forward with Alzheimer's disease includes admitting that a problem exists. When homes are left unlocked, driving leads to tickets, and money disappears, help is needed. Acknowledging the need brings proper diagnosis and supportive information and guidance. Many health issues manifest themselves in ways similar to Alzheimer's disease (agitation, forgetfulness, stress, or depression). A qualified gerontologist or neurologist assures that you receive proper information and advice so that appropriate interventions may be made.

- **Anger** —Anger is a demon of rage and may arrive and take hold of the victim or of the caregiver and family. This anger may be self-contained anguish or it may be something vented on others even when there is no plausible cause for such reaction. Anger often comes and then goes when bits of hope and reassurance appear only to explode in unexpected blasts. Diverting anger into safer methods of dealing with it may help: walking or jogging, building models and participating in crafts, writing and raving and then tearing up the paper and tossing in it into the garbage, or screaming into the wind are tools that have helped me.

- **Blame** – Blame is often tagged to place the fault on someone or something else or even on the individual with Alzheimer's. Sometimes there are errors by doctors, family upheavals, or friends who seem unsupportive, but most often the blame on Alzheimer's brings no positive results. Alzheimer's is not something a victim wishes for or self-inflicts. It is not contagious, although it may be inherited. Steering away from blame clears vision and is essential for renewing a positive outlook. Blame and anger working together greatly add to pain as they reduce the hope for healing and may cause further harm to one's health.

- **Helplessness** – Helplessness often means giving up or falling on "Oh, well, there is nothing I [or anyone] can do." While currently there is no cure, there are some drugs and treatments that are helpful especially with early detection. It is important to remember that the loved one with Alzheimer's did not give herself this disease; it is also important to call for support to escape fugues of helplessness. Whether you are the one with the disease or caregiver, support is critical to well-being.

- **Guilt** – Guilt is the feeling that this happened because of something you did or did not do; this may also extend to the "would have, could have, should have" sensation of regret in "If only I had…"

Children and adolescents often spend great amounts of time in this emotion as do families and friends who have parted from the loved one in anger and have not found or created the opportunity to make up. You are not the cause of Alzheimer's disease. Examining and releasing feelings of guilt build toward a positive attitude that is vital to good health and rebuilding relationships.

- **Regret** – Regret is many times tied to guilt but it also includes feelings of helplessness with less blame on the disease or the death and more blame on good times that could have been if only Alzheimer's had not arrived. Know that good times are possible even under the shadow of Alzheimer's. Regular routines, quiet walks, and avoiding confusion make life seem sort of "normal". Every minute is precious and as times of cognizance become scattered and few, treasure them for the momentary flashes of reuniting that they provide. Regret may also be the wish that you had behaved differently. Since the past is impossible to rearrange work toward a happy now and happier tomorrow.

- **Forgiveness** – Forgiveness means pardoning the disease, your loved one who has passed, the mistakes that have been made, or the difficulties that have arisen. Forgiveness requires time but it brings such relief and clarity of vision for the future. Forgiveness absorbs many negative emotions, empowers the forgiver, and leads to recovery. Forgiveness enhances and revitalizes life.

- **Acceptance** – Acceptance entails knowing that while the long journey of Alzheimer's is devastating, it is essential to move forward. It does not mean you have to forget or that the pain of loss will never return, but it does mean that the world can take on a lovely glow once again. Acceptance helps you surface from the whirlpool of grief to breath wholeness (or near wholeness) once again.

Renewal Resources

There are many tools to help you as you travel through the multifaceted feelings that abound with an

Alzheimer's diagnosis as you search for treatment for symptoms and hope for the remaining years of life. While there is currently no cure, there is abundant hope for a good life within the timeframe that remains. Life will be different and there will be changes but there can be goodness as well.

- Set up an initial evaluation with a physician who you know and trust, and who is familiar with family history.

- Seek the names of respected neurologists and gerontologists who specialize in aging and set up an appointment with one; request an extended appointment so that you have time to share worries, to note changes you have seen, and to learn more about the diagnosis, treatment, and choices for quality care, medication, nutrition, and improved health.

- Understand the profound impact this diagnosis has on your loved one and give her love and respect. Arguments and denial may ensue, but remaining calm and brave help as you work together to find the best health choices.

- Hold family discussions. While sometimes this is impossible due to dynamics, frank conversations before and during Alzheimer's descent build a united front for facing and battling through the disease.

- Allow your loved one to voice his vision, his wishes, his choices, and his requests for health care now and in the future. Sometimes these wishes may be hard to grant as the disease progresses, but early discussions demonstrate a commitment to the best care and sincere concern for the person with the disease.

- Research on-line sites for additional information once a diagnosis is provided. Be wary of any site that makes outlandish promise for improvement. Right now, there is no cure, no prevention, and no reversal.

- Visit your local Alzheimer's Support Group; most communities have outreach programs that meet once a month to offer information and guidance.

- Look for answers to your questions at www.alzforum.org
- Check out clinical trials that may offer you new hope for a cure at www.clinicaltrials.gov

Refer to **Memory Activity #2** (page 135) in **APPENDIX I** *Healing: Reflection and Writing Activities* to support you during diagnosis and as feelings run the emotional gambit for you, your loved one, and members of your family. Reflection and writing clarify intense feelings as they unleash others. Recognizing and managing mental state while enduring grief is beneficial to you and it strengthens your ability to care for your loved one. These help ensure that negativity and stress do not overrun your life. Dealing carefully, honestly, and wisely with the range of emotions that accompany Alzheimer's disease is vital.

Notes and Reminders:

Chapter 3
Circuits that Are Not Circuitous
Navigating the Terrain

Sandra's Story - Decisions with Dad

My brother Bob had called a couple of times to tell me he was worried about Dad. I knew there was a problem with him forgetting things like where his shoes were or how to get to Aunt Jessica's but I just ignored the warnings. I convinced Bob to put Dad on the plane to have him fly out and spend a few weeks with me and he agreed (with that sort of "you'll believe me now" attitude). Unfortunately, Bob was right and I knew it the minute I spotted Dad wandering toward baggage. Formerly an independent, confident man, the old gentleman who funneled along with the mob of passengers toward his suitcase was a shadow of my dad. Without the pressing crowd he may have ended up lost anywhere in the airport or beyond.

I waved and he smiled, but not really at me. He just trundled on. I grabbed his arm and hugged him and after a second he relaxed and that's when I think he recognized me as his daughter. We grabbed his bags and walked out to the car. It was his old Chevy that I had been driving for years and he knew it on sight and smiled. It was nearly lunchtime so we pulled into a café for a snack. Dad ordered pancakes - normal for him as he loves breakfast. But when the food came, that lost look fell over his face again. Then he returned for an instant. He buttered the pancakes, but then looked worried. He reached for his orange juice, eyed it with care, and quickly dumped it over his meal creating a soggy mess.

My first reaction was to scold him but the veil of trouble on his face halted me in mid-word. This was not a joke. A tear formed in his eye and he said quietly, "My mind just isn't working right." Those are the only words he ever uttered to me that suggested he realized he had a problem. He obliterated the idea and disguised his mistake with a smile. It worked for him, I guess. But it made it *harder for me to find ways to help him. I knew doctors and medications might make a difference but his stubborn refusal for help ended that idea. He preferred to slip into silence rather than admit a problem.*

Circuits that Are Not Circuitous
A degree of similarity links between living or witnessing the slow descent of Alzheimer's disease and Enduring Grief.
Abilities, skills, and emotions flash back and forth. One morning breakfast is eaten, the bed is made, and appropriate clothing is worn. By mid-morning, an angry shout, "When are we going to eat?" is followed by all clothing being d as your loved one marches to bed with a solemn (and naked) "Good night!" It is widely recommended to maintain your daily routine as much as possible with meals and activities in scheduled succession. But remember to laugh on those days when a bizarre picture of confusion replaces your "daily routine". Carry on as if all is normal and avoid arguing as a person with Alzheimer's will rarely relent. She is right. Period.
With Alzheimer's there is a disconnection especially with current event, new ideas, and learning. Abilities change: sometimes imperceptibly, sometimes in an instant. What is all right today vanishes tomorrow and then returns later on during the week. It is when the moments of lucidity become brief flashes of minutes or hours rather than days that many people can finally exit denial and enter the reality of Alzheimer's disease.
Early diagnosis is recommended to rule out other possible causes of "forgetfulness" but pinpointing need is tricky with Alzheimer's as good days and bad days alternate; sense and no sense vacillate.

Navigating the Terrain
The following diagram exemplifies changes that are often noted in people with Alzheimer's as they transition from independence to dependence. Remember the progression is the steady loss of memory and skills, but the loss is speckled with returns to seemingly normal behavior. The loss is most often neither sudden nor total, but rather little by little over a period of years. On the bright side, the good

days and good times build strength to face the days where the world feels as if it is falling apart.

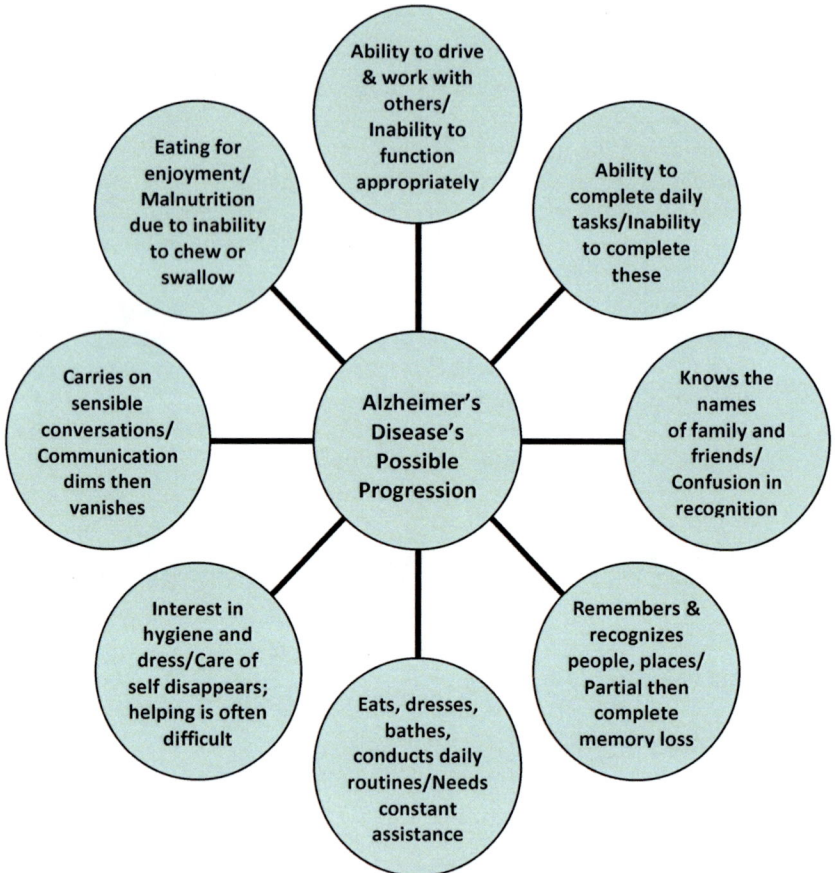

Ability to drive & work with others/ Inability to function appropriately

Eating for enjoyment/ Malnutrition due to inability to chew or swallow

Ability to complete daily tasks/Inability to complete these

Carries on sensible conversations/ Communication dims then vanishes

Alzheimer's Disease's Possible Progression

Knows the names of family and friends/ Confusion in recognition

Interest in hygiene and dress/Care of self disappears; helping is often difficult

Remembers & recognizes people, places/ Partial then complete memory loss

Eats, dresses, bathes, conducts daily routines/Needs constant assistance

I would like to say as I did with Enduring Grief that not every victim moves through each of the above bubbles, but my experience has been that, unless there is early death from another cause, all individuals with Alzheimer's move through these stages until they become totally dependent, unable to communicate, and incapable of primary functions. Alzheimer's disease is often compared as the reverse of the development of a baby. Babies move from birth and dependency to gradual then total independence. Those with

Alzheimer's move from independence to total dependency and death. My greatest struggle with this analogy is that the development of a baby is filled with joy; destruction from Alzheimer's produces profound sadness.

Insight and Understanding

It is a good idea to begin a journal noting the changes you see in your loved one with Alzheimer's to establish a pattern of change. This will also help your physician as s/he makes a diagnosis and prescribes next steps. As one begins taking a medicine such as Aricept or Namenda improvement may be so gradual that you might almost miss it unless you maintain a record. Or there may be little to no change at all. It is believed (hoped?) that medication works positively. However, we do know there is no cure, no reversal, or no prevention.

My stories of my mom and Carole come from dredging past memories. I have spent many years thinking, replaying, and writing about my Alzheimer's experiences and I now recognize so many symptoms that warned me of the disease but that I was unable or refused to see.

Mama developed many coping skills to hide her memory loss. A near car wreck led her to hand over her keys although she never revealed the complete trauma and secrets of her "almost accident", she just stopped driving. She circled the date on the newspaper to keep track of time; she left her television on all day to keep voices flowing through the rooms of her home; she always had cups of red Jell-O ready for grandchildren to appear prepared for guests; and she posted notes to remind herself of upcoming events. The biggest signal of decline came from our conversations on the phone when she adopted a new kitten.

We would be chatting along when she would explode, "That darn cat!" followed by the crash of the receiver and wild commotion as I imagined Mama racing around her living room trying to catch the cat. Sometimes she returned to tell me good-by; at other times the phone just echoed the cat chase and then silence as Mama moved on to something else. When I visited later that month, Mama was covered with scratches and claw marks from the now notorious cat. At that point my sister Judy made the doctors appointments described in Chapter 2 Admitting a Problem.

With my sister Carole I recognized a problem far earlier. While I could not say the word "Alzheimer's" aloud because it held such pain, I realized that Carole had memory problems. She had become increasingly reclusive. While Rich her husband worked, she stayed at home. There were days when she did not say hello to another person until Rich returned or our sister Jackie stopped by after work. She had never really liked television so she did not have that "conversation", she quit reading books, and so it was just her cat and dog that provided entertainment for her during the day. Eventually, Carole lapsed into silence.

Jackie's Story – Hard Changes

It was Christmas when I realized the urgent needs of Carole. I had noticed some behaviors were not quite right, like forgetting to pay bills or getting lost in the store, but the following hit me with a sense of impending disaster. We were wrapping presents together, a task that we had always enjoyed. We both liked to work slowly and meticulously and so our gift-wrapping personalities matched well. Suddenly Carole became very quiet and still. She had a gift tag in front of her with the pen poised, but she sat frozen.

"Carole? What's up?" I asked.

As if in a trance she pushed back her chair, stood up, and walked away from the table. I reached out for the card she attempted to write and saw the beginnings of a name and then a line of ink dragging to the side. She had forgotten how to sign her own name. Later that afternoon Carole asked me to label her packages for her, a simple request with no reference to the previous scene. I filled them out, vaguely acknowledging the seriousness of the problem.

A simple loss, but it marked a tremendous change in our sister. Fortunately we sisters are close; we talk, share laughs, and know we can depend on one another for love and support. To face Alzheimer's alone would be so terrifying. Even though we had different ideas for approaches to Carole's care, we remained a family and that has been a genuine gift. And our dear Carole knew that we loved her.

She good-naturedly tolerated our interventions and sometimes misguided attempts to help her as she patiently taught us lessons of dignity and love.

Reviving Hope

Your journaling routine will help you better understand physical and mental changes of one you noting what went well and what did not. Refer to the following chart as you evaluate changes in:

- **Daily tasks:** Writing a check, letting the dog out the door, moving furniture to set up a Christmas tree can be mind-boggling for an Alzheimer's victim. Look for simple tasks that have become insurmountable projects. Determine if there is growing confusion and misunderstanding.

- **Knowing names:** Many of us confuse names but with someone with Alzheimer's it becomes standard. They might think a grandson is the son or perhaps his/her own grandfather. Argument may ensue over names and events; remember that you cannot win. A nod of agreement is an excellent choice. When sense makes no sense, fighting solves nothing.

- **Remembering and recognizing people and places:** Your favorite restaurant may become a scary place especially if it is dark and noisy. Neighbors may become unknown faces, friends a blur of confusion. It is when recognition of you and close family members fades that it hurts the most. Again a nod of agreement works best; avoiding confusion is helpful and alleviates stress.

- **Eating, dressing, bathing, and conducting routines:** As short-term memory fades it is easy for your loved one to forget if s/he has eaten. Individuals living alone may become increasingly thinner even though the shelves are stocked with food simply because they do not eat. Selecting clothing becomes confusing and so wearing the same dirty clothes solves the dressing dilemma. Showers and baths are noisy, puzzling, dripping, echoing fear

chambers so hygiene declines since baths transform
into traumatic events.

- **Interest in hygiene and dress:** The scary
  bathroom is best forgotten; the selection of
  appropriate dress is also a decision of enormous
  magnitude and so an interest in self-care disappears.
  It can be frightening for a confused person to be
  stripped and stuffed into a shower. A quiet, warm,
  low-level bath with a handheld shower nozzle for
  directing the flow can be soothing. Senses de-
  sensitize so a bathing suit may seem perfect for the
  snow, hat and gloves ideal for summer heat. Unless
  clothing poses a danger such as frostbite in the
  bathing suit, gently offer a suggestion for other
  clothing and then calmly wait for the idea to catch
  hold.
- **Conversing skills:** As it becomes harder to retrieve
  correct terms, silence may pervade. Those with
  Alzheimer's often stop talking because their
  conversation skills are confusing to others who are
  always correcting or filling in the blank or the
  internal struggle to find the right word is just too
  agonizing. Or conversation may become babble with
  incomplete sentences and thought intertwined.
  Even in confusion your loved one has feelings and
  embarrassment hurts. Older adults may also have lost
  their hearing and so people shout or talk slow in a
  way that can be demeaning. Being a part of the
  conversation even though in small snippets offers
  dignity and a sense of belonging.
- **Problems in getting along with others, making
  decisions, becoming angry over small
  misunderstandings, or completing work on
  time:** In early stage Alzheimer's when your loved one
  is still working co-workers may note changes in
  personality that signal potential worries and indicate
  health issues. Sometimes as family members we are
  just too close to "see" a problem and an outsider
  may offer a different view.
- **Driving habits and ability to work with
  others:** One of the toughest decisions is removing
  the privilege of driving. Many police officers receive

training on how to approach and assist drivers with Alzheimer's and they recognize the dangers of their driving, but officers have shared with me that it is difficult to issue a citation to a confused individual and just taking him/her home seems so much kinder, as a ticket is evidence to refuse renewal of a license or to revoke one. Placing the burden on the police is often easier than forcing the keys out of Dad's hand, but sometimes it has to be you.

- **Eating changes:** Meals may be forgotten or when set out may go uneaten. You may have just completed breakfast when your loved one asks, "When's breakfast?" Later there maybe problems using utensils as forks and spoons become mysteries or in separating meal segments: soup dumped on the sandwich, juice poured over cereal. In the late stages of the disease it is not just remembering to eat that creates a problem but the eating itself. The inability to chew may cause a loved one with Alzheimer's to choke. And worse, eventually s/he forgets how to swallow at all. "Failure to thrive" is the term used for malnutrition and eventual starvation that occur to with many late-stage Alzheimer's.

Becoming Whole

A list of such enormity can make caring for someone with Alzheimer's seem impossible. Carole's last few summers at our lake cabin became increasingly difficult. At first it was little things like stumbling into the edge of bed again and again, bruising her shins and stubbing her toes in what became part of her nightly routine. There were incidents like forgetting her towel and clean clothes in the changing house when she headed out to our outdoor shower, which meant that when she was done she had no towel for drying off, and nothing to wear.

Forgetting things once is a reasonable possibility; forgetting again and again becomes a warning sign. Sometimes as these dilemmas tackled her, she mysteriously solved them. At other times they overran her as she stood in bewilderment until someone rescued her. When her "forgetting" became more serious like wandering out into the lake with her shoes and clothes on and never really noticing that she was wet or turning on the teakettle and then lying down for a nap, never remembering that she had started the water at all, we had to face reality. Her cabin visits were about to end.

Another signal came from our traditional game of Gin Rummy. Carole became completely confused about the card game. To avoid having her feel left out we each took turns sitting by her to casually sort her hand into appropriate groupings and help her stay on top of the game as inconspicuously as possible and to let it appear as if the decisions were all her own. During our last game together Carole was bound up in confusion to the point that she could not even hold all of her cards at once; some were held backwards while others protruded awkwardly at odd angles from her hand and a few were scattered on the table in front of her or had tumbled to the floor.

Niece Michelle was gently trying to help her sort out the mess when Carole broke down. At first it was one tear and then another until she was sobbing. Then she abruptly stood up knocking over the high-backed chair, and stomped angrily from the room mumbling angry incoherence. We sat speechless and then we began to cry too. Alzheimer's had become too real.

Renewal Resources

While it is difficult to find or feel renewal as a loved one becomes the victim of Alzheimer's disease, it is important for caregivers and families to work together to support one another. People perceive "reality" differently, through their own lenses on life. Denial is all right until denial becomes dangerous; anger is normal until anger becomes all-consuming. If spouse and children, siblings and significant others can discuss without judgment, the best outcomes for the loved one with Alzheimer's disease and the primary caregiver can be met.

Considerations:

- Should the loved one with Alzheimer's disease reside alone, at home, in a residence...?
- What responsibilities will each family member assume as the not circuitous circuits are encountered?

- What legal issues need to be addressed immediately? Power of Finance, Power of Attorney, medical decisions, wills and trusts...
- Who will assist with paying bills, making payments, completing purchases, and handling money?
- How will run errands like grocery shopping?
- What relationship should be developed with law enforcement personnel for wandering, driving, breaking laws such as the possibility of inadvertent shoplifting?
- What about meals? Hygiene? Care of home? Routines?
- How can a family settle disagreements without severing trust and relationships?

Ideally families have discussed life transitions far in advance so many of the above questions are never serious issues but frequently these discussions are avoided. Later it is left to individuals and family members to interpret the best interests and critical needs of a loved one and that is when problems may arrive.

I do know this: right up to the end of their lives, my mom and sister remained people. While they could not speak, recognize, interact, or demonstrate their love, I know they were there, inside and entangled, but there with me. Remembering their previous vitality helped me better face the painful intensity of decline and death.

If your family is struggling to face this Alzheimer's and conversation seems improbable or impossible, remember you have support from your local Alzheimer's Support Group and/or organization and their hotline: 1-800-272-3900
You are never all alone.

Memory Activity #3 (page 137) in APPENDIX I *Healing: Writing and Reflection Activities* guides your writing for this section. As you write over time you will quite likely discover that you are able to release emotions and inner turmoil with unbelievable freedom. The more you write, the easier it becomes. The easier your writing flows, the more you will want to write. Writing is a safe release during difficult times.
Notes and Reminders

Chapter 4
Facing Baffling Reality
Family Diversity

Carole's Story - Time to Quit Denial

Portland became the setting for Carole's surprise 60th birthday party. Invitations were written and mailed to each sister and niece. Airline reservations were placed and hotel rooms reserved. Dubbed "The Aunt Party", this yearly outing became a reunion custom. We knew ahead of the party that things were "not quite right" with Carole but then again, she still appeared to be functioning fairly independently. I blamed "tiredness" for making Carole seem more forgetful on the phone or confused in the wobbly handwriting in her letters. I had determined that most of the time she was fine as I ignored the possibility of problems. Remaining "denially detached" sheltered me from acknowledgement of significant changes.

As Carole and the San Jose crew clamored up to the hotel desk, she knew us but she did not know us. She recognized us, but did she? We were safe and caring friends but names and relationships appeared shakily unclear. While Carole laughed and smiled with us, dimness trickled from her eyes, unsure of just what was happening.

The next morning's adventures included visiting the Portland Zoo. With a crowd of fourteen it is easy for someone to wander away so when Carole became separated from us in the reptile pavilion, it was not considered a big deal. When she turned left instead of right when she exited the bathroom and then wandered aimlessly for several minutes, that also was deemed as no need for worry. After all in time she had simply circled back around the building to find us just to the right of the exit waiting for her, wondering what was taking so long.

When Carole bought a stuffed polar bear, she had trouble deciding how to pay for it. She counted and recounted her money, confusing tens and twenties, but again we shrugged it off as no problem, just a bit of momentary confusion in a very noisy building. Perhaps the cashier had mumbled the price and that had added to the money mess. Excuses rang out as familiar words; excuses were far better than contemplating the truth. Later Carole set her polar bear bag on a counter and wandered away to another store but again, these things happen, bags are often set down and forgotten. Little "forgetting" when examined individually; big "forgetting" when compounded.

The next big event was the birthday cruise. We arrived at the peer with only minutes to spare (Carole had forgotten her jacket and one cab of family had had to return to the hotel to grab it - funny!). Soon the engines revved up and the diesel fumes filtered into our noses and mixed with the night air as we floated out onto the river. City lights twinkled from the bridges and tall buildings as we made our way, smoothly gliding with the flow of the water. The party was proving to be just the right way to honor Carole.

With dinner consumed dessert arrived. We glanced up as our waitress walked toward us with a special parfait for Carole and her family with one single candle flickering on the top. As I shifted my gaze from the firelight to Carole's eyes, I was struck by the emptiness. Carole half-smiled and half-frowned in confusion as the delicacy moved toward her.

"Where am I? Who are you? What are we doing?" She tried to speak but her words were a muffled mutter as she failed to unravel any sense in the scene. Emptiness stalked our table.

Carole looked alone in a crowd, sad and scared and lost. Who knows what was zigzagging through her mind. Baffled by the in and out, coming and going of Carole, we sang to her, wolfed our dessert, and returned to friendly conversation that circulated the table. Carole remained silent, never uttering another word.

Our sister Judy whispered to me, "Look at Carole. She is having so much fun!" But when I looked, I could not find the fun. I recognized loss.

Facing Baffling Reality

Oh, there were so many signals during that weekend that Carole was not cognitively all right. We recognized them just as much as we avoided them. We tried to adjust to them just as hard as we worked to make them vanish. An "outsider" might have noticed things that we "insiders" simply ignored. When you are close to the scene and it is your loved one, it is difficult to have unbiased vision and clear understanding. And who would imagine that one so young, someone who had just turned 60, could possess so many signs of Alzheimer's disease. Forgetting people, places, and clothing items, not understanding money, leaving purchases behind, disorientation, and so many more confusing events had taken place. But it is hindsight that is the wise teacher.

Family Diversity

Fortunately, even though the four sisters viewed Carole's Alzheimer's dilemma differently we all wanted the best for her and we wanted her to know that we honored her, admired her, and respected her. We hoped that she realized that even in the darkest, saddest moments, we loved her. Clouded mind, confusion, withdrawal, and disengagement never detracted from this.

Most decisions for Carole's care came from her husband, Rich. He retired early so that he could devote time and energy to her care. Although she spent some time in rehabilitation facilities like after she had broken her hip, Rich always just wanted her to come home to be with him. His gentle attitude and forgiving behavior were characteristics of his devotion.

Making decisions for care is not always quite so simple. Your mom may have demanded, "No nursing home ever!" so what do you do when you work, Dad is disabled, and no in-home care is available? Perhaps Grandpa is ornery and cantankerous to the point that the care facility cannot handle him without sedation, and sedation makes him blurry. What choice does a family have?

Imagine children and grandchildren torn apart with decisions for care. Even though Cindy has offered to have Grandma in-home, what about young children if Grandma is traveling through a violent period of Alzheimer's disease? Decisions for care and care giving may strengthen a family as plans for support are shared, when love overrides personal hurt feelings. Discussion and openness are certainly valuable assets when it comes to the care of a loved one with Alzheimer's. Remember too that while Great Gramps cannot always voice his opinion, he certainly has one that flickers ever so briefly to life. Including him as a functioning being in care conversations may alleviate many misunderstandings plus demonstrate love and dignity.

Insight and Understanding

The true revelation of loss came to me from Carole's eyes. Her eyes were open, but the glimmer and reflection of light were gone. This would be something I would see more and more frequently over the next seven years until eventually all of the light would be snuffed into darkness.

After the birthday cruise we returned to the hotel and we helped Carole shrug into her pajamas and snuggle underneath her soft comforter. Not a sound was heard from her until the next day although I have to believe that there were some muffled sobs in her throat. It had been a puzzling day for her, one she could not fully grasp or understand. Fear and joy wound together in a bewildering package for us all as we tried to deny, understand, and accept.

It is hard to know how much to say or and to share with someone with Alzheimer's. Does she really want to have her own fright affirmed? Does he really want his errors in judgment and understanding blared out into the public air? What is the difference between occasional forgetting and frequent forgetting? Have odd habits made safety and security an issue? Or are they just odd habits?

Making decisions for others who appear unable to make them for themselves is an enormous and overpowering responsibility, but by admitting that a problem exists, there are possibilities for making life easier. In the early stages, especially if there is a spouse or other full-time caregiver also in the home, a daily phone call of drop-by visit from children or other family members and friends who care may be enough to allow a degree of relief or reassurance for both the one with Alzheimer's and the caregiver. However, as the disease advances phone calls and short visits are not enough. Even though the caregiver may deny weariness or stress, caring for someone with Alzheimer's (or any debilitating disease) is overwhelming and exhausting. Find delicate ways to intervene and offer assistance. Support might include:

- Lunch out – your treat; hire a caregiver to stand in while the full-time caregiver enjoys a reprieve.
- 2 or 3 hours of respite for the caregiver; you attend to the loved one while the caregiver is free to roam.
- 1 or 2 hours of quiet visiting with a loved one allowing conversation and warmth to radiate.
- An overnight stay for the caregiver with family or friends so that s/he get a really complete night of rest and the chance to relax and revitalize.
- An overnight stay with your loved one by close family or a friend to free the caregiver and allow some personal time with a loved one.
- Housekeeping/yard care assistance; sometimes just having a helping hand with the dishes is a pleasure.
- Shopping or bill paying assistance. Sometimes caregivers are so afraid to leave home in case something happens that cupboards are bare and bills sit unpaid. Look around to see how you can provide help.
- Run errands, buy stamps, and offer your personal service. You may need to volunteer several times before you will be taken up on it.

Sometimes your offers may be greeted with open arms; at other times you may need to be a bit forceful. It is not easy for adults, especially those who have been strong and independent, to accept help either as the person with Alzheimer's or the caregiver. Know that it may not be easy to help adults who have become stubborn, argumentative, and hard to manage. That is when your patience, understanding, and willingness to ignore senseless outbursts and move on as "normal" will be beneficial skills. You may find frustration at nearly every turn but remind yourself of love and dignity and that your loved one with Alzheimer's, though belligerent at the moment, is an innocent victim.

Remember too that caregivers often fear burdening others or they are afraid of appearing inattentive if they do not spend every waking moment caring for a loved one.

finagle some time when you can help and the caregiver can just "go"!

Reviving Hope

While recognizing that there is a problem is difficult and acting on it is almost impossible, a proper diagnosis can clarify necessary actions that will help someone with this disease. Again medications do not cure Alzheimer's disease but they may lessen some of the symptoms making the loss of functions more tolerable.

Nelda, Ralph's wife and primary caregiver - finding and accepting help

At first it was little things like "Where did you put my socks?" or "Why did you do that? I told you not to!" Over time the questions transformed into accusations as if I were hiding things and playing tricks on him.

At first I argued. It was irritating listening to him and each assault made me madder. And then we moved from little things like socks and the remote to things like stealing his money, selling the car, or tricking him into going places like a restaurant with the cruel intent of embarrassing him. It was about to become unbearable when I read about an elder clinic being held in a town near us. Although the examination was just a quick overview of Ralph's symptoms, we received brochures and information that educated us on what the problem might or might not be plus we had resources and a guide to specialists.

From our family doctor to a neurologist and a field of tests we received his diagnosis: "Early Stage Alzheimer's disease" Although these words scared us, we now had some direction. Ralph began a regime of medication that calmed him, we found an activity center where he could meet and socialize during the day, and I discovered a support network for me. At first getting help was difficult because Ralph refused it and he argued about the "nitwit" doctors, but the right medicine has made the last few years better. I refused help as well,

wanting to remain the "perfect" wife and caregiver.
Sometimes you just can't do it all alone.

Becoming Whole

Recognizing and admitting the presence of Alzheimer's disease are steps along the long journey of confusion and decline. Knowing that symptoms may be signs, admitting that a problem exists, and reminding yourself that there is help even with the cloud of Alzheimer's disease offer a degree of reassurance.

Facing reality means that you should receive an appropriate diagnosis, hopefully early enough in the disease to begin a medication regime that lengthens and strengthens cognition and quality of life. It also gives you time to talk with your loved one about his/her wants and wishes. Often Alzheimer's is considered taboo and to talk about it is like wishing it to be true. There are many topics to discuss including health and financial considerations and personal wishes, conversations that when held now may make future tough decisions just a little easier.

Some with the disease and their caregivers may refuse to talk, again because admitting the possibility is viewed as capitulation to the disease. Others do not want to burden children or family with worry and so impending Alzheimer's is neatly hidden from sight, disguised, and ignored. Sometimes open discussions are impossible because of the looming appearance of the disease. After all, who wants to even consider that Mom will become incontinent, Dad will wander and get lost, or that Grandpa will argue and shout at the Senior Center until he is no longer welcome to attend.

Renewal Resources

As our Portland weekend drew to a close we checked in at the airport and headed for security. While security was not as rigorous as we are used to these days, it still required showing identification and tickets. Carole had to dig in her purse until finally she emptied her bag on the counter to find her ID. Taken out for her incoming flight it had been haphazardly tossed back in and lost. She eventually retrieved it, averting a potentially enormous problem.

As our flights were simultaneously announced, we rounded the group with hugs and then fanned out for appropriate gates to the left and right. Suddenly Jackie turned and asked, "Where's Carole?" We glanced around. She was nowhere in sight. We peeked into the lines of other passengers waiting for flights and down the long corridor. No Carole. Nieces raced into bathrooms. Sisters spread out to the restaurants and other airport hiding spots. No Carole anywhere.

We regrouped in failure with fear beginning to creep in. "Jackie, grab your group and head to your flight," I ordered since I had the latest flight. "I'll run to security and get a search going for her. We can't all miss our planes. When I find her, I'll get her to your gate and if it is too late, Allison and I will take her to Reno and then decide what to do next."

Running, calling, and bobbing our heads side to side, sweat boiled as the search drew into a state of frenzy. Allison and I dashed toward security and with increasing panic I shouted, "I've lost my sister!" Then as suddenly as she had disappeared, she reappeared, standing next to two kind ladies — airport angels — who were holding her hands, drying her tears, and reassuring her that everything would be all right.

"You know," one of the angels whispered to me, "when she reached security, we knew something was wrong. It was in her eyes. She was lost and did not know how to be found. So we stopped her from leaving and then calmed her as she started to realize that she did not know what to do. We knew you would come."

Both angels smiled warmly, both knew my fear of the worst. They murmured that everything would be all right and I wished that that could be truth. I realized that things were never going to be "all right" again.

It had taken seven years to reach this point of reality but I had to face reality and admit that Carole was not okay. Things were happening that were out of my control, out of her control. I knew many of the symptoms of Alzheimer's disease, especially the empty, lusterless eyes, the same eyes that increasingly invaded Carole. It would be easier to go on pretending, but that had just become impossible and unsafe, but it would be wrong.

Many signs warned us of Carole's progression but it required a near-calamity to move us into really accepting reality. Again, we worked together in a united effort of care for Carole.

Some of Carole's symptoms included:

- Confusion with getting things out (her ID) and putting them back
- Forgetfulness with gathering items like coats, purses, and keys
- Puzzlement with directions (driving, baking, sewing)
- Trouble counting and converting paper and coins
- Perplexity with scenes like the birthday party
- Difficulties recognizing familiar names and faces
- Problems participating in well-known activities like cards
- Invasion by blank, empty eyes and vacant stares

It is painful to share her symptoms with the fear that you may recognize a terrible truth within them for your loved one. Just remember that in facing the reality of Alzheimer's disease you may receive a diagnosis of a different and treatable disease, or at least ease your mind with correct information so that you can make wise, informed decisions for care.

Memory Activity #4 (page 143) in APPENDIX I *Healing: Writing and Reflection Activities* supports your writing for this section. Thinking, preparing, arranging, and rearranging work best as you plan ahead while remaining flexible to the many potentialities of life.

Notes and Reminders:

Chapter 5
Wandering, Searching, and Losing the Way
Discovering New Paths

Albert's Story - Becoming the Caregiver

Helen and I enjoyed 57 years of marriage before I noticed that she was not doing very well. Maybe the kids saw it first saying things like, "Mom sure seems like she needs a bath" or "Mom is sure weird on the phone these days." I just ignored them, after all they had left home long ago and I loved Helen. I knew I could take care of her and the kids' talk of nursing homes just made me angry and more determined to keep her at home.

Then Helen started wandering. One day I went to the post office. She hadn't wanted to come with me plus getting her into the car had become tough. She was all mixed up. When I got home the front door was open and she was gone. I walked around and called, checked with the neighbors, and then I got in the car and followed some of her old walking routes. Sure enough about twenty minutes later I found her. She must have sprinted to get three miles from home. She appeared confused but also relieved and just a little bit ticked that I had "left her for no reason".

The next week she wandered off again but this time she headed toward the freeway; a few days later she wandered down to the grocery store and wondered why she was there. Then she started getting up at night so I installed locks with chains so she couldn't escape, but she managed to do it anyway. This time police officers found her wandering through backyards. Someone had phoned them. She could have been shot as an intruder. Luckily she had on her silver identification bracelet with her phone number and so they called and then brought her home. Our local police know us, they know Helen has some problems, and they know what to do to calmly coax her instead of scaring her.

Police rides became routine with Helen. Fortunately our city police chief had notified his officers and when she'd go missing I could call for *help or at other times they just recognized her and helped her. She had become increasingly frightened over the last months but these guys knew to approach her in a friendly way, call her by name, and suggest – not force – a ride home. Their kindness worked.*

Eventually I installed an alarm on the door plus I got nighttime caregivers to come every once in awhile so that I could sleep through the night.

Helen's gone now. We laughed and we cried but somehow we got through this disease together. Lots of people ended up helping me.

Wandering, Searching, Losing the Way

Albert's story is one that is common. Many caregivers try to solve all problems on their own, not wanting to bother others or to worry them with the difficulties of Alzheimer's disease. Albert was also fortunate. He had good health and so he was able to take care of Helen on his own. He was also lucky to have an informed police force that cared enough to take the time to keep Helen safe. When area police assume the role of guardian angels, good things almost always happen.

You can also see that through Albert's reflections and his writing, he is finding some peace. No one expects caregivers to survive the death of a loved one and then immediately shift into "happy mode". Healing takes time.

Finding New Paths

After our interview and with many re-readings, Albert's story touches my heart. Brave spouses demonstrate amazing strength and the power of giving to a loved one who has Alzheimer's. Albert tried to talk with his children but they were not ready to listen to his needs and not ready to understand his stress or his wishes. This lack of understanding is understandable: we each view life (and death) differently. We perceive good choices from our own perspective and it is often difficult to incorporate our belief of what is right with that of others. There had been family anger over the locks, the wandering, the police intervention, but Albert had found ways to make his life with Helen safe and secure. Caregivers take the role of angels in many forms.

The primary caregiver of someone with Alzheimer's sees him/her daily and often misses digressions just because these become a way of life. Forgetting the directions to the grocery store one day is backed by a successful shopping trip the next day so problems can be ignored, if they are even viewed as problems at all.

"Outsiders", and I am including anyone who lives outside of the home or who visits the less than once a week, may see changes as enormous signals of inability that more frequent visitors miss or they may just deny that there is a problem. We must be gentle as we share our observations and not shout them. Most caregivers cope as best they can and often do not recognize or want any other alternatives or interventions. kind insight and input may help.

Insight and Understanding

Each day caregivers face a tough job as Alzheimer's disease shapes and reshapes the behaviors and abilities. Realizing and accepting help may be hard to imagine as requests feel like impositions. Most people who offer help mean it; most people who help once are willing to repeat the service. Some possible requests include:

- Inviting friends and family to stop by frequently to visit, observe, and interact (in a gentle, non-forceful ways).
- Accepting help when it is offered; this can be difficult for independent caregivers who do not want intrusion of any type.
- Sharing personal convictions as to the proper way to handle this very difficult situation while acknowledging that other approaches might work as well.
- Listening to sincere advice and input from others while recognizing the final decisions will most likely be your own and those of your loved one when s/he can still articulate them.
- Avoiding promises that may lead to feelings of guilt later on, i.e., "Yes, I'll always keep the farm" when the work and stress become unbearable or "No, I'll never resort to a full-time assisted living facility" when falls, dangers, and illness make home care unfeasible and unreasonable.

- Accepting respite breaks for time alone or to complete errands; most people who offer time and help really want to assist you.
- Installing locks or alarms on doors to prevent unexpected "escapes" or a adding a bedside alarm pad.
- Notifying your local police when you believe there might be a problem with wandering.
- Purchasing an identification bracelet with first name, "Alzheimer's disease", and a phone number to call for help. Avoid putting an address since unscrupulous villains may prey.
- Researching tests, trial studies, and medications that may make a positive difference for you.

Reviving Hope

A few months before my mom died my daughter Allison and I cared for her for a week so that my sister Judy and her regular caregivers could have a vacation. Mama was down to a speechless routine of wandering up and down her hallway. She would sit down for a bite to eat and in the evening I could coax her to bed, but otherwise she paced incessantly. She could no longer take care of personal hygiene so toileting and bathing were wrestling matches we undertook with stress for me and fear for her.

Throughout that week the only time I left her house was to race to the mailbox and back or to sit on the porch so that Allison could play in the yard. Mama would not come outside and forcing her was impossible. It was a good week because I was with my dear mother, but it was a sad week because my mom was void of life and understanding. Then suddenly on the last day as Mama strolled by me she paused, glanced at me, clapped her hands together once with a jumping gesture she had always executed to show her joy and said, "Oh! I am so glad you're here." Then in a flash she returned to her blank stare and endless tromp.

It is hard to explain how wonderful, how warming these words and gesture felt. I often recall that brief moment when my mom knew me and it reminds me that even in the deepest throes of Alzheimer's disease there existed an inkling within my mom of who I was and that I loved her. That is one reason why when I hear people say that "Mom is oblivious" or "Grand-Dad is completely out of it and doesn't care", my heart disagrees. No, it is not as it was before, but there is still a thread of connection. I know this is true because I have lived it.

Becoming Whole

Becoming whole may seem absolutely impossible, especially in the mid- to late-stages of Alzheimer's disease when abilities are stripped away, never to return. Even having traveled this journey twice with family and several more times with my support group members, the pain is fresh. Observing the day-to-day dying of one you love consumes the spirit and drives away feelings of hope and optimism. Here are some suggestions that may help you endure the pain and remain strong:

- Replay happy events and family gatherings in your brain
- Recall sweet sayings and beautiful gestures to remind you of love
- Be prepared for every possible angle of confusion; this will save additional angles of confusion
- Decide what you can and cannot do for your loved one:
    o Bathe and dress
    o Cook, share meals, and/or feed
    o Attend to toileting
    o Converse and make the senseless make sense
    o Shop, clean, and attend to household needs
    o Manage finances and correspondence
    o Schedule and transport to medical appointments
    o Provide transportation as needed
    o Address critical medical decisions
    o Maintain your own health while devoting hours to the health of someone else
    o Preserve patience and understanding under disturbing circumstances
    o Avoid anger
    o Ask for help when you need it
    o Accept help when it comes
    o Decline bothersome interference

Some people willingly attend to all of the above; others may find that they are comfortable with none of them. An open discussion, as free from judgment as is possible, solves or resolves many worries and stresses involved in taking on the responsibilities of long-term care of someone with Alzheimer's. It is also important to remind yourself to appreciate the honesty of others and what they feel they can and cannot handle. Share your own concerns. Honest and open communication prevents many negative side effects.

Often you will find that another family member can complete items that you cannot. Teamwork when it comes to care lessens the burden as it strengthens family bonds. Not always – some people do not bear up well under such tremulous conditions but others rise to new heights of helpfulness and understanding.

I was fine with every aspect of caring for my mom and sister from bathing to feeding to clipping nails to driving to appointments. But changing dirty pants was horrible. It is hard to comprehend that as a caregiver for those who had cared for me I had to do things I never imagined possible. But I did it. They needed me for the most personal of care and I knew I had to respond to their call. Stressful, embarrassing, nauseating, yes, but sometime we are braver than we have ever dreamed! Caring for others develops wonderful characteristics in you, characteristics you may not have imagined you possessed.

Renewal Resources

Your local police department along with your support team may be willing to help you with personal concerns that you have for a loved one. This may include:

- Writing tickets for traffic violations. I imagine that caught you by surprise but if Grandma's driving is getting scarier and she somehow manages to renew her driver's license, a ticket can wave a warning flag to the issuing agency. Police can step in to prevent driving where family members may be stymied by the reluctance or refusal of a loved one to stop.
- Writing citations for infractions such as shoplifting or jaywalking. Lack of moral judgment may tell Mom to just pocket anything she needs at the store. The goal

of a citation is not to end Mom's freedom, to send her to jail, or to embarrass her; the goal is to protect her. Predators may be watching her, noticing changes in her behavior, and noting her inconsistent judgments. More eyes watching over her with care are reassurance for her safety from the eyes of those who seek to deceive and harm her.

- Keeping an eye out for your loved one as s/he takes his routine walk. Many people walk with the same pattern so a thoughtful officer or dear friend can be on the lookout in case confusion arises and the walker becomes lost or if the walking route drastically changes and leads the wanderer into danger.

- Ordering an identification bracelet or watchband that says the wanderer has Alzheimer's and a phone number for contacting help. Do not put the victim's address; again predators may lurk.

- Installing a home alarm system to warn of unscheduled or unexpected exits, especially those that occur in the middle of the night.

- Installing a phone alarm system that is voice activated if your loved one needs help. Those with early stage Alzheimer's may sense a problem and call for help. Caregivers can use the system to get assistance when needed.

- Calling for assistance from law enforcement in case of violence or threats. People with Alzheimer's may become violent, swinging and hitting, wielding weapons such as guns or knives, or making wild threats. Police officers can help to calm and recommend professional sources for help or require professional intervention that may include a neurological examination or short-term care in a licensed facility to determine the best medications and health assistance.

- Creating stick-on nametags with your phone number that you can gently attach to a jacket or back of a shirt in case of separation. The tag often must be stuck on surreptitiously so that the victim is not embarrassed by the tag or angry because of your well-meant intervention.

- Designing small cards to hand out in case of a public scene or uneasy situation. It simply states:
  Patience, please.
  My loved one has Alzheimer's disease.
  This little card can circumvent and alleviate misunderstanding from gawking crowds or misguided observers who stand in horror when your loved one is in distress.

- Digging into reserves of resourcefulness, strength, and resiliency that support you through the day, the week, the Alzheimer's term.

As we delve deeper into Alzheimer's disease, you may begin to feel that there is no hope and the road ahead will be nothing but crushing. I do not mean to frighten you with grim stories and harsh warnings, but being equipped with knowledge and helpful hints saves you from the stress of feeling isolated and powerless.

You are probably starting to recognize a pattern of angels with people with Alzheimer's. Regardless of your religious and spiritual beliefs, I think you will start to realize that there are good people everywhere, people who are ready and willing to assist you. Some know you personally; some are friends of your loved one. And then there are others who come out of nowhere just when you need them the most.

The Sisters' Story - Remembering Connections
After one of her surgeries Carole had gone to a rehabilitation facility not far from her home so that she could have around-the-clock care and to relieve Rich as caregiver. When we visited we loved to bundle Carole into a warm sweatshirt and pants and then lift her into a wheelchair for a roll out onto the patio and into the pleasant wintry California sun. Carole enjoyed the fresh air, the gentle breeze, and the calming atmosphere outside of her small, stuffy room. Somehow a silly phrase from childhood slipped into the conversation, "Well, bless his old bones!" At the sound of these words Carole started to giggle. A smile beamed across her previously empty face as she mumbled words beyond

our knowledge. Then she resumed her silent stare. Surprised by this connection, we soaked in the joyous moment that had brought Carole back to us for just a flash.

Many times that afternoon the phrase worked its way into our chatter, and every time, Carole emerged from the depths to giggle. This angel phrase let us escape the tragedy of her disease for seconds and reminded us of her definite presence with us. I wonder what she was thinking. This is such a warming memory.

I believe that even in the most devastating depths of Alzheimer's disease, somewhere within lies a flicker of life, a connection, a sense of love. **Memory Activity #5** (page 144) in **APPENDIX I** *Healing: Writing and Reflection Activities* directs your writing for this section. It has been said that we truly grow in knowledge during the toughest of trials. Think about this as you write. I know you will find bits of truth in this concept.

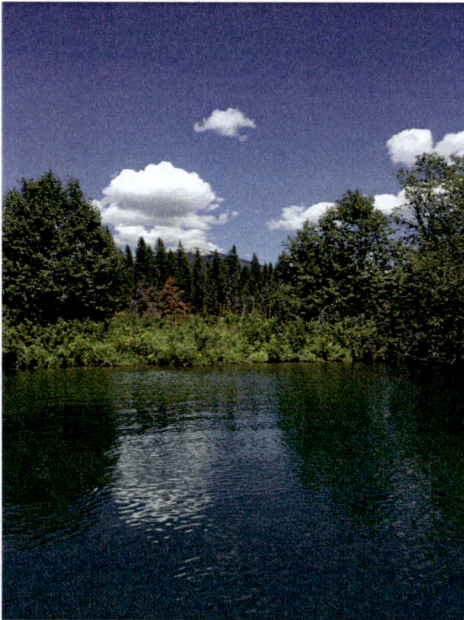

Notes and Reminders:

Chapter 6
Going Places, Eating Out
Remaining Connected

Carole's Story - Family Excursions

We never wanted to leave Carole out of anything we were doing, although I suppose that sometimes our expectations for her were unreasonable. But pretending she and we could handle it perpetuated our illusion of Carole whole again. The following two tales detail our last two dinner outings with family. We learned from them both and both experiences changed us, expanded our understanding, and increased our connections.

A favorite eating spot is Buca di Beppo, a fun-filled restaurant not far from Carole's home. The size of our group never mattered as there are alcoves and side-rooms to accommodate any celebration. By the time of our last dinner there, life for Carole was very puzzling. I was settled in at the opposite end of our table of seventeen with Carole far away at the other end when Rich signaled me to "Come".

"I think Carole needs to go to the bathroom," he whispered. Even though she wore adult diapers at the time, we still tried to make her habits "normal" so I grasped Carole's hand and she willingly followed me. We wound through the labyrinth of many dimly lit, chatter-filled rooms and hidden corners until finally we reached our destination. Carole was agitated as I shoved the heavy black door open and her agitation soon intensified. It was even darker in the restroom than it had been in the restaurant and this unfamiliar "cave" emitted a rather musty odor.

Over the loudspeaker above the sink an Italian voice jabbered and shouted, accompanied by tinkles of non-descript piano notes and bursts of brassy horns. The discord added to the sinister atmosphere as the bathroom mission transformed into a nightmare. Carole wrestled to escape from me as she muttered a series of indistinct words. Her

70

eyes searched for the exit as I pleaded with her and yanked her back into the room. She relented slightly so that I could maneuver her into the stall, twist her around to face me, and reach back to lock the door.

Dark, noisy, and smelly, Carole was getting angry. To add to her plight I pestered her by grabbing her waistband and pushing her pants down as she tugged and struggled to pull her pants back up as she mumbled unfriendly words. The harder I pushed the more determined she became at hoisting them back up. We fought like this for five minutes – an inch down, an inch up, two inches down, one inch up - until I finally got them below her knees and out of her reach. I felt a small sense of miserable victory but Carole would get the best of me yet.

Now I needed to get her to sit down on the cold toilet seat tucked away far below her. I gently wrapped my hands around her tiny waist and forced her downward. She locked her knees and refused to budge. "Please, Carole, please. Just try to sit down." Well, of course, my pleas fell empty as the guttural guffaws of the blasting speakers enveloped us. I pushed and pleaded but Carole remained flexed and immovable. She had firmly taken her non-cooperation stance. I had won the pants battle but I had not won the bending war!

Dripping frustrated tears I finally said, "I guess you do not have to go. Let's give it up."

She sort of sighed through her anguish and mumbled, "Good!"

I tugged her pants back up her legs and reached back to unlock the stall door so that we could exit. Of course at this instant the toilet self-flushed, adding whirling racket, flying water droplets, and scariness to the scene. I once again clutched Carole's hand, reassuring her that the torture was about to end and carefully guided her out of the stall. Washing her hands at the sink was simply out of the question but I scrubbed my own as she headed for the door. Fortunately it was heavy and difficult to drag open so I completed my cleaning job, grabbed a wet towel for wiping her hands, and then helped her out. We trundled until we rediscovered our family who awaited our return.

"What took so long?" several shouted as I tried to steer Carole to her former seat. I smiled limply as I pointed out Carole's chair to her and indicated that she should sit down. Surprise! She refused to take her seat. Again she locked her knees and remained stiff as I shoved and I begged. Carole ignored me as her eyes shifted to the far end of the table and she began to stumble her feet into motion. Knowing she would win again I asked, "Carole, would you like to move down to the other end with Christi [our niece]?" She instantly began to shuffle her feet in that direction. This time instead of pulling her along behind me I assumed the pushing position with my hands firmly planted in the center of her back. Carole didn't seem to mind and so we "choo choo trained" our way to the opposite end of the table and prepared for Carole to squeeze in.

I plopped down in my chair, pointed to her new chair, and patted the seat. "Here you go, Carole. Sit down." Blankly she gazed at me, then at the chair, then at the two booths behind us. In one booth there was what I label the "Young Lovers". In the other booth sat the "Gawkers", a middle-aged couple whose mouths hung open as they surveyed our complicated travail. Carole eyed one table and then the other until she made her decision and headed toward the Gawkers. This couple did not appreciate their in-coming guest although the man acted as though he sympathized with our plight. His wife, however, donned an evil scowl and thrust her purse into the empty space on the seat that Carole was trying to fill. I mumbled apologies, grabbed Carole's hand, and tried to drag her away, hoping to avoid additional cruel glares.

As I pulled one way, she pulled harder in the opposite direction until she broke free of my grasp and lunged closer to the Gawkers. The woman's face became ever-more threatening and she pushed her purse further out on the seat and brushed her hand in the air as if to shoo my sister away like she was a fly or scary bug. The gentleman looked on sadly but also helplessly.

It was at this moment that the Young Lovers, having witnessed our struggle, called sweetly, "Here, she can sit here!" The inviting voices redirected Carole's attention just long enough for her to relax and take a step away from the table of misunderstanding and toward the table of kindness. Two angels were willing to reach out to strangers in need, signaling their acceptance of my sister.

Carole hesitated as she turned in the direction of the Young Lovers and then took a shuffling step toward their booth. Then she pivoted slightly and spied her own family anxiously waiting for her to rejoin them. Carole stared with what appeared to be blank eyes, but she somehow recognized that there were two chairs that needed bodies at our table, my old one and the new one set for her. And then it finally dawned on me. She just wanted to be allowed a choice, to make the seating decision on her own.

"Which chair would you like, Carole?" She glanced left and right and then chose my former chair and quickly tumbled in. I wedged Carole and her chair as far underneath the table as possible to prevent any attempt at flight and quickly filled the seat next to her. Our dinner was laced with laughter and with tears as we realized that our attempts of inclusion caused more pain than joy and our meals out with her would soon end.

We did undertake one more dinner at the Cheesecake Factory. Fortunately on this occasion we were assigned a table that had a long vinyl booth-like seat on one side and chairs on the other. Five family members quickly filled the chairs, as the rest of us slid into the booth, Carole included as we toppled her in. Since her pants fit her very loosely because she had lost so much weight I grabbed a handful of cloth on her pant leg and pulled her toward me as I scooted further in along the bench. Then Jackie sat down and pressed in next to Carole to shove her until she was snuggled *tightly between us. She appeared content, wedged between two loving sisters.*

The best part of the evening was dessert. There were ten of us and we each ordered a different type of cheesecake. Once all ten slices were in place we each took a bite in unison, chewed slowly as we savored the rich, creamy delight, then we rotated our plates clockwise around the table. As plates arrived in front of each diner, we scooped up the next tasty bite of a new flavor dessert. While Carole needed assistance loading her spoon each time, she smiled as she enjoyed every nibble as the plates paraded around the table from start to finish. This dessert rotation has remained a tradition that reminds us - happily - of Carole.

Going Places, Eating Out

These two stories combine to make a very long tale, but there are so many signs, signals, and lessons that needed to be shared. It is rather fantastic that our last two meals out have created such clear, poignant memories for me. I learned about my family, outsiders, the good and the bad, myself, and more.

Going places and including a loved one with Alzheimer's are rewarding experiences just as they often create troubles. As you read on you will discover many ways to make trips and restaurants pleasant experiences rather than distressing debacles. One thing to remember is that each visit away from home is different. While it may be the same diner with the same menu and familiar clientele, to one with Alzheimer's the scene may take on a menacing aura. The regular menu may be confusing; friendly faces may appear mean; chatter and an ambient noise may become clatter and thunderous disruption. If agitation is invading and escape seems the only logical plan, leave. Meals can be boxed, excuses can be shared, and most people will work to help you, just like the Young Lovers. Gawkers do not understand and must be relegated to the far reaches of life.

Confusion may also occur when visiting someone else's home. When "I want to go home" becomes the only comment of the day you have a couple of choices. Say, "Yes, soon" and redirect the conversation as many times as you and your loved one can tolerate or simply defer and go home. Do not be surprised, however, if after you leave, your loved one asks why you left so early when you were all having such a fantastic time.

Remaining Connected

And through all of the challenges with Carole and with Mama, we remained connected to both of them and connected to one another as a family. Those who could not bear to see the devastation visited less often than those who could face it. Those who were willing the change dirty pants and give showers did so. Those who could not perform personal duties found other ways to help such as:

- Assistance with grooming and dressing
- Cleaning the house
- Washing, drying, ironing clothes
- Shopping for food and for other necessities
- Cooking meals
- Taking loved one and caregiver out to dinner, for a walk, to the theater...
- Offering respite care
- Running errands
- Driving to appointments
- Offering extra listening ears with doctors and medical professionals
- Sitting and listening, engaging in conversation, and spending time in peace

Your gift of time can make a wonderful difference.

Insight and Understanding

Maybe Carole did not really know where we were or whom she was with, but she did know that adoring people surrounded her. What Carole could not do, we did for her. What she could not say, we tried to fill in the blanks without overwhelming her while guessing at what she wanted to communicate to us. Though escape from the sticky threads of Alzheimer's disease became shorter, she was very much with us in heartfelt ways.

There are lessons every day in caring for a loved one with Alzheimer's disease. Some lessons strike at a moment when they are clear and understandable, like forcing Carole into her seat at the table. Of course she wanted a choice; she was an adult, had feelings, and had preferences. I shoved her into so many bad spots again and again but the seat at the restaurant was the incident that finally hit me, "Let Carole decide." Of course, if there is danger, you must make the choice, but when possible let him/her make it.

Familiar spots like a favorite restaurant can become a frightening ordeal. Re-evaluate dining out with considerations such as:

- Is the restaurant bright and cheery? Darkness breeds fear.
- Is the restaurant crowded? Crowds cause confusion. Perhaps select a dinnertime that is off-peak so you still enjoy a preferred dining spot minus extra people.
- Is the restaurant noisy? Loud, distracting noises add to agitation and confusion. Rethink your eatery.
- Will your loved one feel safe and secure when you dine there?
- Are the waiters and waitresses helpful and understanding or are they rushed and impatient? Select places that cater to you and your loved one.
- Are there chairs that you can slide far under the table or booths where you can wedge your loved one in to prevent the desire to wander?

Bathrooms are another important consideration. I know you cannot always check the restroom out first but it may be a good idea. Again you want a room that is well lit and quiet with a large stall for two people. One of the biggest problems that is not fixable is a crazy flushing toilet. Some flush at the least movement so spewing water may sprinkle a loved one who is already wary and tense. Another problem is low seats. I think the person with Alzheimer's feels as if s/he is falling into a pit and of course a frightened reaction transpires.

Clientele is another consideration. No, you cannot enter and ask grouchy people to leave but you can search for a section that has friendly faces that exude welcome. For some reason there is a group of people who believe that dementia and Alzheimer's are contagious or something your loved one has wished upon him/herself. Fortunately, most people are kind and empathize with the situation. When you sense desperation and know that you are about to break, pause and glance around. Quite likely there are angels who are ready to help you.

Reviving Hope

With foresight and planning you will be able to continue many of your favorite routines. Again thinking ahead for possible problems and offering choice make a tremendous difference. Trusted friends and family may want to accompany you on these outings. Include them when they are helpful and patient; exclude them if they are negative or if they in any way make the trip harder or more stressful. After all who cares how Granddad is dressed as long as you feel his hygiene needs are being met (Chapter 7 Hygiene, Personal Care, Maintaining Beauty). Who cares if Mom eats with her hands or only wants dessert as long as she is safe with you? It can be problematic and maybe embarrassing when behavior is slightly awry, but if there is enjoyment, continue to relish every moment of joy that is possible. And sometimes even the most distressing situation will be laughable later on. Keeping a sense of humor is essential as an Alzheimer's caregiver or family member.

Sometimes as the caregiver you need time alone. Perhaps Tuesday you'll take your loved one to lunch and then on Thursday you might ask a neighbor to sit in while you take an hour or two for yourself. I worry constantly about those with Alzheimer's. I watch horrified as ability after ability vanishes. But my experiences make me very aware of the caregiver, too. Caregivers need support, tender help, patience, the opportunity to vent without judgment, and the affirmation that others care. Friends and family, please offer help knowing that this may be refused (repeatedly) even when it is needed. Also realize that your point-of-view is different from anyone else's. Share insight and advice, but without negative force. Most caregivers are under enough stress and distress; they do not need more.

Caregivers, remember that friends and family understand as best they can and they offer assistance accordingly. They are not in your shoes in the daily routine of your life. They have ideas and solutions that most often are well meant (even though they may not be well received!). Bravery and stamina are critical caregiver traits but you do not have to do it all alone.

Becoming Whole

Think back on a familiar routine or favorite adventure that evokes happy memories. Use it to replace clouds of sadness, worry, or frustration. The dessert rotation with Carole will be one that we institute again and again as it is fun, delicious, and makes her feel near.

Gerald's Story - My Dear Ellen

I never thought our lives together would end in the way they did. Ellen always took care of me. She packed my bag when I traveled; she prepared nearly all of our meals. She always let me choose the restaurant, our vacation spot, and the brand of our car. I don't think she minded, but I wonder now if maybe she did. I'll never forget my first trip after she died. Who would pack one shirt, three pairs of slacks, and no sandals for a vacation in Hawaii?

What I miss most are our evenings together. Ellen had gotten to like her glass of wine each night. We'd sit out on the porch, rock in our rockers, and watch the stars. It isn't the same without her at night but I try. Sometimes I fill two glasses of wine, one for her and one for me… just in case she decides to join me.

Again it is time and reflection, distance and healing that make Gerald's story one of hope. There are second guesses and wondering, and there is the deep sense of loss, but Gerald is finding ways to carry on his life. Caregivers, remember that there is life after loss; family, remember that those who remain need your love and tender care. Call, write, or visit to help survivors survive.

Renewal Resources

While eating out or traveling may never be the same with a loved one with dementia, it can still be rewarding. The biggest difference is planning ahead for:

- Quiet locales with soft or no music
- Good lighting so that scary possibilities are gone
- Menus that match eating habits and abilities
- Chairs that prevent a getaway

- Staff that understands and appreciates you and your loved one
- Bathrooms that are well lit and quiet... you know what I mean!
- Toilets that do not self-flush at inappropriate and unnecessary moments

You can create note cards with the message:
Patience, please.
My loved one has Alzheimer's.
For most people a gentle reminder such as this is adequate. One time Carole and I were on a trail hike when a herd of wild bicyclists descended upon us. They called out, no, they yelled out, "Get out of our way!" Of course, my sister ignored them (she may not have even heard them). I reached for her hand as they shouted again and she stumbled toward me. I responded to them gently, "Please. My sister has Alzheimer's. Do not shout at her." Their faces changed from anger to sorrow. They dismounted and carefully and silently passed us. I hope they learned a new way to behave.

Memory Activity #6 (page 145) in APPENDIX I *Healing: Writing and Reflection Activities* channels your writing for this section. The activities invite you to recall good deeds, great angels, and happy events that brought joy to you when you most needed it. There is also a tiny spot for devils, the inconsiderate and thoughtless people you may have encountered during the Alzheimer's journey. Glancing back prepares you to move forward.

Notes and Reminders:

Chapter 7
Personal Care
Maintaining Beauty

Carole's Story - Appearance Concerns
Another aspect of Carole's decline was in self-care, her hygiene and personal attention and clothing choices. She had begun to pace nearly non-stop which caused her shoes to fall apart as they transformed into a walking disaster. The tread wore smooth, seams unraveled, and they flopped around on her feet like wild geese flapping in a windstorm. Along with the shoes, Carole's hair had taken on a life of its own. Rich cared for her and protected her but there were things that The Sisters noticed as "girls" that remained insignificant to him. She'd always been slender but now her metabolism and eating habits had changed her wardrobe into baggy pants and stained shirts. Formerly elegant clothing now appeared like discarded rummage sale items tossed on an unwilling and disinterested scarecrow.

On one visit I decided it was time to step up and make some changes for her. I picked up a phone book and started reading addresses to Jackie who was familiar with the area in search of a hair stylist nearby. Angels steered Jackie's choice to The Stylist and a quick call resulted in an appointment with Lily for a shampoo, trim, and set. We combed Carole's hair down from its stand-on-end position, found a clean shirt and pants for her, located "cute" socks, and then thrust her feet into her tattered shoes.

Getting Carole out the front door and into the car had become a battle. If we did not catch her early she would turn away from the door and return to her indoors wandering. Once we had steered her outside we had to maintain guidance right up to the open car door as she liked to climb into the car backwards with feet wedged into the crevasse in the back seat and her body scrunched against the front seat. Untangling her presented a unique problem because as soon as we tried to adjust her body parts, she became stiff and

80

immobile. Coaxing, shoving, and patience settled her with seatbelt snapped so that we could head out to our destination. Once we arrived another wrestling match ensued as we extracted her from the car for the stroll across the lot to Lily's. Pleading mingled with frustration but finally we had both of her feet on the ground and we pulled her up and out, problem solved for the moment.

As if by innate sense, Lily recognized us and met us at the edge of the sidewalk. She gently grasped Carole's hands between her own, kissed them warmly, and slowly guided her into the shop and onto the waiting chair. Lily shook out the cape and wrapped it carefully around Carole's neck, all the while murmuring soothing words meant just for Carole. I whispered to Lily, "She's sometimes confused – she does not know what we are doing." I couldn't say the word "Alzheimer's" as it was too horrible to utter, so I skirted the term. Lily nodded and replied, "I know, I know. But she is safe with me."

Lily knew Carole by instinct and her kindness brought peace. Lily's loving care felt extraordinary although it was ordinary for her. She soon had Carole looking marvelous once again.

After Lily completed her work we guided Carole to a shoe shop next door. Her favorite shoe style was on display in the window and the shop conveniently prevented another into/out of the car adventure. The saleslady greeted us warmly. I pointed at Carole's shoes and asked for a similar pair since they fit well and would be familiar to her. The saleslady replied, "Well, take a seat. We'll have to measure her feet." Futilely I explained to unhearing ears that it would be easier to just guess her size and go from there, but the saleslady insisted that that was impossible as she determinedly pointed us to our designated chairs. I guided Carole and persuaded her to sit down, catching her slightly off-balance so that a soft push landed her in her chair.

As I gently wiggled Carole's shoe to loosen it from her foot, the lady returned with her shoe-

sizer stuffed under her arm. She stood in front of us tapping her toe impatiently. As I worked harder to get the shoe to release from her foot, the clerk tapped a little more loudly with staccatoed impatience. "Please, can you just bring me a shoe that looks about like this?" I pleaded as I pointed at Carole's shoe. "No!" came the unspoken reply displayed across the clerk's unyielding face. Her friendliness had vanished.

Finally Carole's foot popped out of the shoe, ready for the next steps of the sizing ordeal. I pointed to the faded numbers inside of her worn shoe to no avail. I then had to scrunch her wavering, bent-toed foot onto the silver shoe-sizer, balance foot and sizer and guide all of this tangle onto the floor while convincing Carole to stand up for a proper measurement.

Imagine yourself, confused and sensing the dislike of someone in front of you. Think about having your foot unwillingly extracted from your shoe and forced onto a hard metal surface. Picture being compelled to stand on this hard device while someone poked around at your toes and heel. Not much fun and quite a tussle! We weren't exactly disagreeable customers but I guess with our ridiculous struggle we were not adequately cooperative either.

After a minor skirmish, the saleslady determined a "9 ½" (faintly written inside the old shoe) and she arose in a huff and headed to the storeroom. Crashing and mumbling echoed from behind the wall and then she emerged with several shoes of many sizes and colors. She shucked the stack onto the floor in front of us as she backed away to busy herself elsewhere in the shop. Ignoring us made our job easier as the pressure of her distaste exited the scene. We rummaged through the pile until we found the appropriate shoes: same color, same size, same style and thus no confusion. Just what we had asked for!

With her new shoes on, Carole stood up, smiled, and shuffled toward the door as we quickly paid and raced to catch up with her. Wearing her new shoes home saved us another painful scene of trying to get her new ones off and her old ones back onto her feet, plus this allowed us to deposit her dilapidated pair in the trash.

Why didn't we just leave that store when our clerk acted so rudely? Well, with dementia you learn to pick your battles: one thoughtless clerk or climbing into the car, driving around searching for the right shoe place, unloading again, entering a store, and perhaps meeting the same degradation as we had already faced, all to get Carole some new shoes. We chose to suffer and fortunately we also ended up with shoes and some tips for next time.

Several months later when again I was in town we drove Carole over for her regular hair appointment and then we re-entered the shoe store for another round. This time we knew the size and felt better prepared for the shoe purchasing process. Fortified by Lily's love and care, we grasped Carole's hands and walked by the large picture windows of the shop and geared ourselves up to enter. When our "friend" spotted us, she ended all eye contact, bent over to avoid us, and then slunk away into the backroom. A young man emerged as the apparent result of a shove as he stumbled into our faces. He appeared pleased to see us and he quickly found shoes that fit by following our simple request. No sizer, no frustration, no disgust. An angel guarded the store that day and he took care of my sister, but there may have been a devil lurking in the backroom as well!

Personal Care

The love from Lily filled us with hope; the disgust from the surly saleslady filled us with despair. Once again we had encountered a kind and caring angel who helped us with dignity and grace. Lily could see Carole as a remarkable individual who had had a rich and delightful life. Maybe it also took the unfriendliness of another to help us better understand kindness and to realize that some people are simply not very nice.

Caring for a loved one with Alzheimer's includes many decisions and choices. When possible, and after time, I learned to let Carole have a voice in the choices. It is an easy deal to ask what another individual wants or does not want and while the response may be confused or not fit into the current need, silent, tender prodding coupled with dignity helps you accomplish almost anything.

Whenever possible purchase similar items of clothing and shoes to save confusion and the statement, "These are not my pants! I want MY pants!" Pull-on pants, shirts with buttons or loose necks, and comfortable shoes that do not flap around on the foot are my suggestions. Hair care and trims are best done in a familiar atmosphere with friendly stylists and little noise and confusion. Just getting out of the door and into the car is enough struggle for one day.

Fortunately those with Alzheimer's generally get out of the car much more easily than they get in. The caregiver may be exhausted but the loved one is usually content to be back home.

Maintaining Beauty

The last night of Carole's last trip with us to Priest Lake I decided that Carole should get a shower before her trip home. As cleaning Carole had become one of my designated duties, I gathered her shower items, clutched her hand, and guided her out of the cabin door and into the breezy, cool forest air. We had an outside shower located a few steps from the cabin, perfect in the daylight with individuals who understood the purpose and pleasantness of the shower routine. Unfortunately it was dark and although tiny moonbeams peeped through the towering trees, it was dim for the job ahead. Plus mysterious forests at night are sort of scary anyway which added to the ever-increasing stress I sensed in Carole.

Carole let me lead her right up to the shower door before she refused to take one more step. She could not see well since I had removed her glasses, it was getting colder, she felt confused, and the dripping water of the shower added to her bewilderment. Nothing made sense and she felt frightened and so she balked. I tugged her toward the shower and when she didn't budge, I stepped behind her and pushed as she strained backward into my arms. I knew that I could force her over this last hurdle and into the warm stream of water with a few more shoves but I was beginning to wonder at the worthiness of this task.

I cried, she cried, and I begged pitifully, but she refused to lift her foot and step into the shower. I yanked on her leg, trying to make her knee bend, but my repeated attempts and pleas wafted into the night. When I was about to give up, she suddenly lifted her foot and stumbled into the drizzling water. My extra force was fruitless until she decided to enter the shower when it finally became her idea to do so. As I nudged her further under the showerhead, she dodged to get away drawing me deeper into the misty spray. We engaged in a water-sprinkled tug-of-war, accomplishing little other than frustration and soaking me more than her.

Carole struggled more as I dabbed suds and shampoo in her direction until we reached a point where it seemed best to simply give up and let her travel home only slightly scrubbed with soap residue on her skin as a lasting sign of my pathetic effort. Just then I heard a tiny tap on the side of the shower, "Can we help you, Aunt Gini?" came the words of my great-niece and great-nephews, Kjelsey, Kaare, and Colin.

"Oh, yes, please," I begged. Kjelsey climbed into the shower with Carole and me and together we grasped Carole's arms and drew her under the warm water as we took turns cleaning and rinsing her. At our sides, Kaare and Colin handed us the essentials as needed – soap, shampoo, washcloth, and finally a fluffy, dry towel. Three more angels had arrived, these three darling children who loved their Great Aunt Carole. They had never known Carole as the vital, adoring Great Aunt, but they loved her just the same and even through the shrouding clouds of dementia, she loved them in return.

That incident told me much about those three young ones. Their kindness and genuine desire to help will never be forgotten. I also know that Carole knew that love was in the air around her that night. Their love helped us survive another traumatic ordeal.

The final shower I gave Carole is one of humor. The Sisters planned a sleepover at Carole's so that Rich could have a break. I was chatting and shared with Marilyn the struggle that had ensued the last time I had bathed Carole – tears from shampoo, soaking wet floor and me, and Carole grappling with me on every step of the job. "Maybe I can help," Marilyn proudly announced.

The three of us headed upstairs to complete the showering task. After cornering Carole in the small bathroom, we tugged off her clothing piece by piece. While the getting out of the clothes was met with its usual resistance, it was evening and time for a slip-over-the-head nightgown so the getting dressed end of the job would be far easier. The three of us managed to then squeeze into the tiny space between the shower and toilet as we set out to get Carole into the shower and under the waterspout. I slid the shower door to the left, adjusted the spray nozzle, and wrapped my arm around her shoulders while giving her a gentle shove forward. Surprise! She refused to step over the tiny ledge and into the shower. When I tried to pick up one foot to lift it in she locked her knee into a rigid stump. I could not drag this unbendable leg off of the floor. I wiggled it and joggled her foot but Carole had dug in, frozen in place. I tried the other foot with a similar result.

Marilyn and I tried begging and we tried pleading, again with no success. We finally laughed and in unison sighed, "We give up," and so Carole stepped first gingerly and then happily into the shower without further hesitation. Her stubbornness and strong will had not yet been totally figured out by us. She may have been out-of-control of herself but she was definitely very much in control of her sisters!

We wormed Carole around until we had her centered under the splashing water. After some calming words and a bit of time in the gentle spray, she settled down and seemed to enjoy the flow of the warm water across her chest. We breathed relief until she suddenly started to twitch and mumble. Not knowing what to do we tried to pacify her with reassuring words as we continued the cleansing job. She twitched some more and agitation started to invade. We cajoled as best we could, rubbing her arms and stroking her face. Then Carole calmly reached behind to her rear end where she gathered a handful of feces. She proudly offered this to Marilyn with a crooked sort of grin. "Here," she said.

"Ack!" Marilyn and I screamed and then we burst into tearful laughter. Only in the throes of something so horrific could laughter release us from the agony we both felt. After a thorough rewashing and rinsing, we turned off the water and patted Carole dry. As we slipped her nightie over her head, Marilyn whispered, "That was awful. Without each other how would we ever get through?"

Sometimes finding humor in the deepest pain allows for healing. This story is the perfect example of that. Losing control of one's bodily functions in an individual of such grace and modesty was beyond words or comprehension. Laughing helps us even now.

Insight and Understanding

As always there are many lessons learned from the shoe and hair ordeal and the showering charade. Some of the lessons were pleasurable, like finding angels who were waiting to step in and help; others caused pain but we learned something every time. Personal care and hygiene can become a never-ending challenge. Even getting hair trimmed can be frightening and overwhelming if the right person, a Lily, is not there to assist you. Lily was gentle, kind, and she reassured Carole that everything would be all right. As Carole's patience wore thin, Lily moved us from the long perm process to short wash-and-wear cuts. Her pedicures (that alternated with my nail clipping sagas) moved from the full works when Carole could still climb into the "big" chair and plunge her feet into the basin of warm water to gentle snips and tender foot rubs when the chair mounting job became an obstacle. Lily found ways to attend to Carole without force or fear.

The shoe sales taught us how different people deal with those who do not understand. Even though our first lady was anything but kind, her replacement worker offered Carole dignity as we purchased new shoes for her. Even when Carole no longer knew or cared about her appearance, her sisters did and they found ways to maintain her beauty. What a gracious (and stubborn) teacher Carole was.

As for clothing Carole had an enormous closet stuffed with outfits, although over time many of her clothes became too large for her tiny body. As Alzheimer's progresses many lose their appetite so eating is another struggle and often they just forget to eat or they metabolize differently so pounds disappear. Maintaining a healthy weight is not easy. We eventually helped Rich clear out the closet so that it contained just a few choices that were close to her size, clothing that was easy to pull on and to remove. Struggling with dressing is no way to start or end a day.

Reviving Hope

It is terrible to watch a loved one who has been elegant and lovely fade into shabby disorder. That is why The Sisters' help for Carole seem so valuable. Caregivers, there are people who are willing to help you; accept their help so you can have some moments of reprieve. A strong healthy caregiver is vital and exhaustion from constant attention to your loved one is a danger.

My brother-in-law Rich was wonderful to Carole. His patience and understanding go beyond any words that I could ever write. Never during the fourteen years of Carole's Alzheimer's descent did I see him angry or hear him utter a mean word. Amazing is the only word I find that matches the love of Rich for his darling wife. We were fortunate that Rich tolerated our "sisterly interventions", things that just required our touch. Haircuts, shoes, and showers were three of our specialties. I think that Rich recognized our good intent, although he may have been quite happy when we left to go home.

The Sisters helped as we could and how we felt that we should but sometimes help can be seen as interference as well. For example, I kept commenting on Carole's weight loss. I understood it came from metabolism changes and her tiny appetite. Rich received my comments of concern as "You are not feeding my sister enough!" I knew that he constantly worked to do everything he could to convince her to eat but forcing Carole to do anything that she had not determined to do was nearly impossible. Little sandwiches and snacks always rested on the corner of the counter so that Carole could grab something whenever she strolled by. As the disease moved forward this worked far better than trying to get her to sit at the table and manipulate a fork or spoon.

Even in the dimmest, saddest hours Rich always said, "You know, Carole and I are still having fun!" It was difficult to see that "fun" but it was simple to see his love and devotion.

Becoming Whole

There are many hygiene needs to be concerned with when caring for someone with Alzheimer's. Some of these are solved quite easily with planning and foresight; others are more difficult because what works today may become a complete disaster tomorrow. Just when you think that bathing is under control, life change. Ingenuity is a necessary companion for a caregiver:

- Dressing and undressing - Sometimes a favorite shirt is demanded every day even when it is soiled or worn out. Wash each evening, if possible, to be ready for the next day, or purchase several of the same item so that the familiar is always available.

- Dressing and undressing - These procedures are exposing, cold, and can be frightening. Try to understand how having clothes tugged off or shoved on can be a scary ordeal that makes no sense. Find slips-ons when possible and make dressing a regular routine: breakfast, dressing, going on a walk, for example. If the one with Alzheimer's puts on the "wrong" items or dons them backward or inside out, who cares? Save the struggle as you plan for tomorrow.

- Getting ready to go some place - Plan ahead and insert extra time. You will be getting yourself ready and your loved one as well. Arrange for any eventuality - weather changes, confusion that forces the trip to be cut short, individuals who may impede your departure or various parts of your trip, and "accidents". With time a loved one with Alzheimer's forgets bathroom skills. A change of clothes (sometimes several) and clean-up products are vital components of your travel bag. Adult diapers (oh, how I am bothered by that term) are handy and helpful but some with Alzheimer's still have a shred of remembrance and wearing a diaper is not acceptable. Some brands are scratchy on the skin and noisy when the victim moves - how irritating and uncomfortable! And they are very expensive which may stretch a budget. Worse to me is that even in the depths of the disease there are internal signals that diapers are inappropriate. Alas, there may come a time for you when there is no other choice.

- Getting into and out of the car - It sounds easy but the car can be confusing. Many families tell me that their loved ones climb in in all sorts of directions and rearranging them can quickly bring on frustration and the end of hope for an outing because anger and agitation now rule. A couple of tips including getting your loved one to sit down and then you help him/her pivot in or guiding the inside foot onto the floor before the other foot sets him/her in reverse.

- Hair care – Locate a hair stylist or barber who overflows with patience. Haircuts and shampoos can be intimidating as an unidentified individual clips, snips, snaps cloths, pushes heads into sinks, and then hauls out buzzing clippers. Short, easy hairstyles that can be washed and then left alone save frustration and struggle.

- Shoes, pants, shirts, and other apparel items – Familiar clothes are familiar. Seek slip-on shoes or loose fitting styles with ties, pants that slip on and have elastic rather than snaps, buttons or zippers, shirts with wide openings for getting over the head, pajamas that fit comfortably and slide off and on with ease, jackets and shirts with buttons or snaps. Zippers sometimes zip skin and clothing creating another caregiver quandary.

- Clipping finger and toenails – Again this can be frightening. It is not easy to grasp a finger, force the nail under a clipper, and then to snap down without cutting skin producing blood or bringing on agitation. Clipping is another sort of personal invasion but it is essential to complete so that nails do not become ingrown or dangerously long and sharp. After a shower or bath is a good time for clipping since nails will be more pliable. But if the bathing has been excruciating, save clipping for another time.

- Familiar items that may become irritating or upsetting:
    Hair spray – noisy, smelly, and strange
    Soaps and shampoos – even familiar brands may emit smells that disturb the victim
    Fingernail polish – irritating to look at on formerly plain nails; the smell during application can be bothersome
    Detergents and fabric softeners that have a strong odor – fragrances can be irritating or produce allergic reactions

Clothing and shoes — easy-on rather than
items that have to be forced on
Trips— just getting out the door can be a
hassle. Sometimes it is easier to just remain
at home.
 Remember that socialization and getting out are
important to well being for both your loved one and you.
Careful planning can make the outing a terrific and positive
event.

Renewal Resources
 A necessary struggle for personal hygiene is bathing.
It is sad when Grandpa emanates odors that rankle the noses
of guests. How sad that visitors avoid your loved one because
Grandma stinks. The smell is terrible, but the degradation of
uncleanness may be worse. Plus being dirty, especially in
personal areas, can produce health hazards. Bathing and
showering become needed evils. Tips for bathing and
showering include:

- Daylight instead of darkness; being able to see helps
  ease and erase some of the fear of the dripping noise
  of the water and scary feeling of the task
- No tear shampoo instead of the stinging type
- Avoiding soaping the face where foam can get into
  the eyes and sting
- Warm, soothing water flow from a removable,
  handheld showerhead rather than water from a
  permanent fixture. This way you can juggle the
  showerhead to reach every spot instead of juggling
  the person around in the water.
- Quick but gentle action for cleaning and rinsing — the
  faster the better, in most cases
- Have clean towels and clothing ready as soon as the
  shower ends

 Bathtubs work well but one problem is rinsing if you
do not have a removable showerhead. Plus sometimes the tub
is just plain scary — it echoes, your loved one is naked and
so feels exposed, getting feet over the tub edge is tricky,
and it is a long way down from standing to sitting and a
long way to stand back up at the end. A shower chair can
be a useful tool.

Showers work well but if the water splashes too hard, too suddenly, or too hot or cold, cleansing may become a nightmare. The removable showerhead and a shower chair are wonderful allies.

Facing Alzheimer's disease is tough as roles reverse from big sister guarding little sister to little sister stepping in as a caregiver. For some reason, while the role reversal hurt because I knew that this disease only travels in one direction, it also gave me the chance to repay Carole for the love she had showered on me. As a challenge and a nightmare, there were also soothing rewards in discovering that I had capacities for caring that I did not fully know existed.

Memory Activity #7 (page 148) in **APPENDIX I** *Healing: Writing and Reflection Activities* guides your writing for this section. An extensive checklist helps you prepare for many of the angles and sidesteps of caring for a victim of Alzheimer's disease. There are also reminders for care for the caregiver.

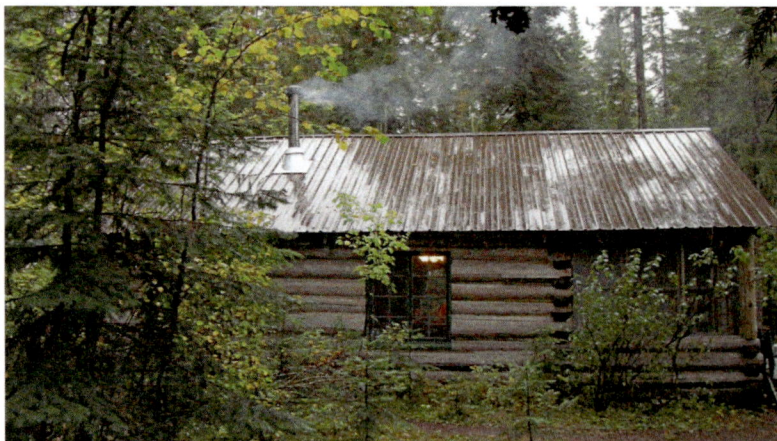

Our Cabin at Priest Lake

Notes and Reminders:

Chapter 8
Indecisive and Difficult Decisions
Seeking Peace

Benjamin's Story – Changes in our home

You can often tell when a woman is no longer living in or taking care of a home. This was very true of Mom's home. The home exuded less and less classiness as Mom slipped further away from her awareness of its upkeep, further away from us. The house lacked her graceful touch and charm.

The most noticeable change was the lack of change. The gold carpet, once so stylish, now lay faded and out-of-date. The dark kitchen cupboards accompanied by olive green appliances again set the house off as outdated. Windows became spotted with water and dandelions snuck in-between the cracks in the sidewalk. Even though Mom and Dad still lived there and upkeep continued, the house lost part of its appeal, its beauty, and its life without Mom's vitality. It felt shut in, shut up, and lonely without her devoted attention.

Piles began to sprout up throughout the house: all of the bills that needed payment, magazines left unread, old newspapers waiting to be opened, and junk mail that accumulated by the day. Heaps gathered dust and created tripping dangers and the only uncluttered spot was Dad's television chair where he spent the evening and a chair that Mom plopped into although she rarely filled it for more than a fleeting moment.

Mom's wandering was intense as throughout the day she drifted up and down and in and out, circulating the house, mumbling and humming as she paced. She never rested for more than a few minutes before resuming her march. She had unknown places to go, places where she would never arrive, but she relentlessly searched for her destination nonetheless.

During her final year slight physical changes became apparent. Her left shoulder began to droop slightly and her pacing reduced to a counter-clock-wise oval in the family room. Doctors speculated *that this was the result of tiny strokes that were invading her, leading to the creation of her lean and loop.*

Her nights became more restless as well. While Mom might doze off with little struggle, it was impossible for her to stay asleep or in bed for long. Dad got up ten, twenty, or thirty times each night. As the disease progressed I knew we needed to hire someone to watch over Mom so Dad could rest.

Indecisive and Difficult Decisions

Watching a loved one deteriorate is a horrible sight. Sometimes it is the person him/herself as s/he forgets hair care and hygiene and at other times it is the disintegration of formerly important jobs. Caring for a home, tending to the grass, paying mounting bills, or simply grocery shopping may become astronomical and so avoided tasks. It is sometimes these external signals that relay to family the critical urgency of family discussion for interventions.

Caregivers, too, need care as much as the loved one who is suffering. They fill an essential role in guarding a loved one, solving problems as they arise, and providing other family members with a sense of relief that all is well. The job is exhausting and sometimes overwhelming. Caregiving becomes a 24-hour responsibility and so other duties fall by the wayside.

Seeking Peace

In an ideal world everything would be timed to perfection. Mental and physical abilities would end at the same moment, everyone would always agree on every issue, and there would be no worries or concerns about anything. Pure bliss would reign. Fortunately (under most conditions) our world is imperfect, thus allowing us to be truly human. Some people live independently right up until the last days of life. With Alzheimer's disease, however, there are months and years when the victim is unable to make critical life choices. A family discussion including your loved one when the initial symptoms of Alzheimer's first appears may alleviate much stress later on. If the victim can clearly articulate her wishes and if the family is willing to listen to and then adhere to them, personal and medical choices can be easier.

Not that discussion solves everything – life is too unpredictable for that – but discussion can help a family in times of crisis.

For example, "No heroic measures" to save a life may be your loved one's wish, but a child might refute the decision and demand feeding tubes and a breathing machine when it is beyond hope that these will do more than extend life for a few days or weeks. With such a situation, family members may be at odds as to what steps to take next. What does Mom really want? What end-of-life decisions does Grandpa really want us to follow? Do not get me wrong. These discussions are hard and heavy; the decisions are even more overpowering. But openness in advance may save family dissolution in the future.

Alzheimer's choices are never black and white. As with any serious decision there are hundreds and thousands of shades of gray. The following are several possible situations/discussions that a spouse, caregiver, or adult children might have with a loved one about extended care:

- *Let's get a complete diagnosis from a qualified gerontologist/neurologist to rule out _ _ _ _ and determine if _ _ _ _.* This is an important first step and is the best step if an appointment with a qualified doctor who listens and cares is scheduled, meticulous examinations are performed, careful diagnosis that rules out infection, illness, or stroke as causes of mental decline is provided, and when a plan of action for medication, care, and overall support for the loved one is implemented.

- *Let's put Mom in Golden Acres. She is definitely not all right and it is wearing Dad out. I think if we pool our resources we can do this.* This could be best step if an appointment with a qualified doctor who listens and cares is scheduled, meticulous examinations are performed, careful diagnosis that rules out infection, illness, or stroke as cause of mental decline is provided, and if Dad and Mom are a part of the conversation and they agree that this is the appropriate course of action. Now Mom may be at a point that she cannot communicate her wishes but what if, somewhere within the clouds of her mind she is aware, shouldn't she know about decisions that will drastically alter her life?

- *Let's let Dad keep Mom at home like he has been. We need to all take turns coming to stay with them to relieve Dad and help with Mom. Dad could use some time off and maybe a vacation. We can do that.* This could be best step if an appointment with a qualified doctor who listens and cares is scheduled, meticulous examinations are performed, careful diagnosis that rules out infection, illness, or stroke as cause of mental decline is provided, and the family rallies to help Mom and Dad with support and kindness. This can be very difficult when one child wants this and another wants that. Arguments rarely solve problems and they often only make them worse. Also when the kids come to help they need to help, not criticize, complain, accuse, fight, interfere, or blame. They need to listen, learn, and offer support. Mom and Dad deserve this.

- *Let's move Mom and Dad closer to use so that we can keep an eye out for them and help more.* This could be best step if an appointment with a qualified doctor who listens and cares is scheduled, meticulous examinations are performed, careful diagnosis that rules out infection, illness, or stroke as cause of mental decline is provided, and Dad and Mom are in the conversation. Moving can be nice, especially a down-size with less cleaning and upkeep. Moving can also be confusing, frightening, and horrible if parents are now more isolated and alone with old friends far away, children busy working, and familiar places and faces gone.

- *Let's let Joey take care of it. He was always the favorite and he lives three doors down. He's been checking on them for years anyway.* This could be best step if an appointment with a qualified doctor who listens and cares is scheduled, meticulous examinations are performed, careful diagnosis that rules out infection, illness, or stroke as cause of mental decline is provided, and if Joey agrees to this additional responsibility **and** if the siblings concur that Joey has authority to make critical decisions. It is difficult enough to step in as caregiver for parents in this role-reversal scenario without Joey being also forced to have every decision second-guessed.

- *Let's just wait and see. Maybe things aren't as bad as they seem.* This could be best step if an appointment with a qualified doctor who listens and cares is scheduled, meticulous examinations are performed, careful diagnosis that rules out infection, illness, illness, or stroke as cause of mental decline is provided, and if things really are fine. When children live close by they can check in and check up often; if, however the children are scattered across the country or if there are no children at all, it could be exhausting, dangerous, and impossible for life to simply continue as if everything were "normal".

Insight and Understanding

Becoming the caregiver for a spouse or parent is a complex mission. It may be viewed as an assignment, a job, a responsibility, a duty, an obligation, or a loving act of kindness (and sacrifice). As you have read, coming to an agreement that a problem even exists may be difficult; the decisions beyond this are much harder and these decisions tend to grow. That is why it is so important to get a proper diagnosis from a qualified physician before determining the next critical steps in care and to keep communication openly with family members.

When determining the caregiver's role remember to consider all of the ways you will be able to help, all of the ways that others may be able to help, and all of items that will be impossible roles for you or for others to fulfill. After all if you are working in a demanding career, if you have small children, if you live far from your loved one who needs care, or if you have thousands of additional responsibilities, there are not enough hours in the day for you to serve as *Super Human Being.* Recall the list of items that included bathing, cleaning, shopping, dressing, and driving (and more!). Are these responsibilities that you are willing and able to complete? Also consider other helpers:

- Children – yours and those of other family members
- Extended family members

- Friendly neighbors
- Best friends
- Home health care resources
- Bonded, in-home health care workers
- Assisted living facilities (from independent, to semi-independent, to skilled nursing)
- Meals-on-Wheels and other home meal delivery systems who also serve as informal "check-in-on" providers
- Activity centers that offer daycare for those with Alzheimer's and other dementias
- Respite care for hourly, overnight, or weekend stays so that the caregiver has some freedom

There are many tasks that spouses and children can attend to or help with; there are other situations and items for which you may need to request outside or additional assistance. Help is available in many forms with a little research and a few phone calls. It is all right for you and for others to say "Yes!" just as it is all right to say "No."

Sandy's Story - Moving Mom

Mom had long ago discussed her end-of-life wishes. She had explained to the five of us that when she could no longer lived alone because of potential dangers (leaving burners on, inability to pay bills, leaving doors wide open, etc.) she wanted to move to Archwood Manor, an assisted living to skilled nursing care facility nearby. We all agreed right up until "moving day". Then my siblings pointed their fingers and said, "It's your decision. You and Bob [Sandy's brother] can take full responsibility. We think Mom is doing just fine." A difficult decision was made worse because my family waffled at the move, although it had been Mom's choice.

We moved Mom and since we could also take along her favorite chair and bedspread, she appeared happy and the care providers seemed kind. Living far away and with Bob and me exhausted from constant worry about Mom, we knew we had made the right choice. I hope that eventually our family will understand, heal, and forgive.

Reviving Hope

The entire scene of decline is horrendous. How do you stand by helplessly as a loved one degenerates in tiny steps as well as through giant leaps? And Alzheimer's disease feels like it lasts forever with its slow progression interlaced with slight glimmers of hope that things are not quite as bad as they appeared to be yesterday.

The following stories offer insight and understanding based on the experiences of other caregivers, family members, and their loved ones.

Grace's Story - the Activity Center

Aunt Grace's house had two sentinel chairs placed in front of her large picture window. She and Uncle Ross could often be seen sitting there, peering out at the world, waiting for company to arrive. When Uncle Ross quit his job to care for Aunt Grace and then lost his driver's license because of seizures that made driving dangerous, the two of them became so isolated. We all tried to help out but our schedules were so nuts and Uncle Ross was unwilling to ask for help. He felt caring for Aunt Grace was entirely his responsibility.

Then we found out about a tremendous service in our community, OutReach. What had appeared to be the end of independence for them both, was solved by a van service that picked them up, took them to the store or to the doctor, and even drove them out for lunch and then returned later to pick them up and bring them home. It was inexpensive and dependable and made them both happy and sort of free.

One day Aunt Grace was reported by the driver as "Incorrigible". You have to know that my aunt was anything but incorrigible. In fact she was so kind we had to laugh that she would ever stir up trouble. I guess one driver had tried to force her into a seat and in her Alzheimer's haze she refused and hit him with her fist and then kicked the seat and huffed all the way to the store. Uncle

Ross begged for forgiveness and pleaded for them to be allowed back onto the van, promising to make her behave. Lucky for us, she has been good ever since!

Check out what your community offers and discover the health care and other services available to help you as you care for your loved one. Share this information with others who may feel they have to "go it alone" when there is potential help in many forms.

Gordon's Story - Susanne's Activity Center Experience

Susanne and I had planned to travel and visit out grandkids after I retired. I loved my job and just could not separate myself from work. In fact I'd still be working except that I needed to care for Susanne. At first she just had little problems like finding her clothes and accusing me of hiding them, or saying she had paid the bills and then a late notice would arrive and I'd find the bill stuffed behind the television set with a scribbled, indecipherable check wadded beside it.

I hired a lady to come in a few hours each day to be Susanne's friend while I was at work. They laughed and took walks but then Susanne became ornery. She started swearing – something she had never done – and arguing about everything. She'd refuse to get dressed or she'd be dressed and then disrobe in the kitchen. She accused our helper of trying to steal things or to poison her.

I wound up my job and took on full-time caregiving. Things went along pretty well for three years as I knew Susanne and her routines and I had learned not to argue. I'd just nod and agree and then redirect the conversation. After all who cared what she wore at home? Who cared if she ate breakfast with her hands? Who cared if she walked up and down the stairs all day and all night? The kids came and helped and she always grinned when the grandkids came by although their noisy play increasingly agitated her. We just worked on quiet *activities and the family helped out by going along with this.*

Then our son Peter began hounding me to get help. Well, it wasn't really hounding, I know he meant well, but he kept on telling me I needed help. Luckily he never mentioned nursing homes; I wasn't ready for that. We were still having mostly good days. But Peter did help me find a local activity center. A bus came each morning to pick Susanne up. Oh, at first I worried about her being angry about going and then sitting with all of those confused dementia folks for the day, but she loved it right from the start.

I rode with her that first day to ease her into her trip. The attendants at the day care greeted us at the door, welcoming Susanne warmly as they guided her to the main daycare room. She hardly looked back at me. It was hard to leave her but I needed to give this a try. This free time let me mow the grass, buy groceries, and straighten up the house without worrying about Susanne. And Susanne transitioned well into this new routine. She'd get up in the morning to wander but once we had breakfast and I got her dressed, she sensed she had places to go. When the bus would appear on our block she'd head for the door and off she'd trundle. I am lucky my son forced me to get some reprieve.

Becoming Whole

Love and care of another individual require enormous reserves of strength on good days; on rough days the strain may become unbearable. The loved one with Alzheimer's may lash out to the confusion and bewildering conditions of the disease and the caregiver may sense that s/he is the intended target. But really, most often, it is the disease that causes the rage. The attacks hurt and so it is essential to remind caregivers that it is the confusion that masks sense and this allows explosions to occur. It is rarely the direct actions or reactions of the caregiver that create the wrath. Remember, however, that although most loved ones with Alzheimer's are guarded with loving care, there are cases of elder abuse, people who harm victims for power or money.

If you find yourself in a dangerous situation with your loved one, it is critical to call for help from the police or emergency care personnel. An extended stay in a facility may be recommended where a complete diagnosis and medical work-up can be completed. There are medical professionals who can help rebalance tempers and thus daily living. Never put yourselves in unnecessary danger.

Colleen's Story – Seeking help as Ben's caregiver

Ben had always had a bit of a temper but Alzheimer's disease seemed to aggravate it beyond his control. He would become inflamed over nothing although he always had an explanation for his behavior. The final blow came when he pulled a gun on me. I knew I had to take action and so I called our local police department.

The officers arrived within minutes and subdued Ben and they worked to calm me, to reassure me that calling for help had been the appropriate action. Through their efforts Ben was "committed" to a 2-week stay in a facility where they ran tests and eventually diagnosed Ben with mid-stage Alzheimer's disease. They started him on some medications to calm him and within days his pleasant disposition reappeared.

An added relief was that when Ben returned home, he had forgotten the outbreak and he had forgotten the forced hospital stay. There was no blame shot at me for "sending him away". Even now, three years later, the police officers that helped me check up on us every once in awhile. That is nice.

One of the benefits of attending a support group or using the Alzheimer's hotline is that you will find kind individuals who listen and share, who understand your stress as you care for a victim of dementia, and who offer sound advice.

Gretchen's story - Dealing with Michael's anger

Michael and I had shared forty-five years of marriage when he became outwardly aggressive to our grandkids. He'd always had a hot temper and over the years I had learned to avoid it, to hide from it, to pretend it was normal. Physical abuse, no, but he was pretty cruel with his words and threats. Alzheimer's disease seemed to release his inhibitions, his check on his behavior. The grandkids liked to stop by after school to stay hi - I'd always babysat them and loved them all so much. I laughed at how they noisily crashed into our house, raiding the cookie jar for snacks.

At first Michael just grumbled about the "@$#^" kids and he'd wander off to his shop or the backyard. Then he started yelling at them and using profanity. One day he grabbed Jacob by the arm and shook him. I stepped in and stopped him but Jacob was scared and didn't understand Grandpa's attack. When I told his parents that was the end of Jacob's visits to our house after school. It nearly killed me but I understood.

So I just started meeting Jacob at the gate as he walked by on his way to or from school or I stopped by his house for a hug and to give him his favorite oatmeal cookies. The doctor adjusted his medicine and that eventually calmed Michael although he still had a mad demeanor much of the time. It was hard not to resent his behavior that caused the loss of the grandkids but I loved him and so I guess things worked out all right.

Sense of no sense? That is Alzheimer's disease.

Renewal Resources

And here I repeat: Caregivers fulfill a tough, unrelenting role in caring for the health and well-being of those with Alzheimer's. Often this task falls to a spouse. At other times children take on this enormous responsibility. It is fortunate when a family can discuss the crisis openly, especially if this discussion can take place during early stages so that your loved one can offer some input and insight and express his/her wishes.

Unfortunately this conversation may be pocked with problems. I list some of them here so that you can weave them into your particular situation and into your family discussion. Information to guide your Alzheimer's decisions includes:

- The loved one refuses to admit that there is any need for worry so critical assessment and diagnosis are delayed when medications and counseling could make life easier.
  Reason and beg, let your loved one know that you too are searching for answers and a diagnosis to help improve your loved one's health. A thorough examination may rule out Alzheimer's disease, not just rule it in as the cause of decline and memory problems.

- A caregiving spouse or significant other refuses help or refuses to recognize the huge job entailed with caring for one with dementia.
  Offer assistance again and again and when it is accepted celebrate; when it is refused try new angles such as delivering hot meals, mowing the lawn, or simply stopping by to listen and offer your friendship.

- Finances do not permit in-home health support or medical treatment.
  Talk to social services or a financial advisor who may know ways for you to get the help you need. Contact your local Alzheimer's support group or call the hotline. Chat with your physician about programs that offer in-home assistance.

- Children disagree on the level of care needed or the appropriate interventions that could be beneficial to both parents.
  Talk calmly and if the discussion rolls toward arguments stop and regroup your thoughts or perhaps disband for today and try another day. Try again so that all decisions are in the open. If conversation is impossible, continue to work as best as you can to keep your loved one safe and comfortable. Tough decisions are heartbreaking and without support they are even tougher. Find a friend who listens to you, who is non-judgmental, and who gives advice only when asked.

- Children and family members live at a distance and so visits, help, and support are limited.

*Try to keep communication open to let everyone know
how the victim is doing and how the disease is
progressing. Find local agencies that offer the sorts
of services that make caregiving easier. Remind
yourself that just because family cannot find ways or
will not take the time to help, it does not mean that
they do not love you both.*

- Children live in different states so that legal
documents like Power of Attorney are not valid if the
parent were to move closer.
*Contact a lawyer who specializes in elder law. State
laws for the care of the elderly vary. Legal advice is
important to insure that correct decisions for care
are made.*

- The loved one has chosen paths and arguments in life
that leave her isolated and alone.
*Even ornery people deserve love and forgiveness. I
read once that to forgive does not mean to forget
but it does mean that you have accepted the
situation and have managed to move on. If the loved
one is truly friendless, support groups and hospice
agencies often provide in-home care. No one should
suffer and die alone, regardless of how she has lived
her life.*

Nicole's Story – My Mom Sarah
    *It sounds trite but Mom always loved my
brothers best. When we were little they had their
own rooms and I slept on the floor; she always
attended all of their ball games and she forgot my
graduation; she doted on their children while mine
just got a card to mark a birthday. I'd always
tried to stay in contact with phone calls and
letters but I also distanced myself from her
criticism and tirades.
    Then Jeff called to tell me Mom was falling
apart. I knew she had been slipping since Dad died.
Her voice on the phone was often wavering and
confused and she sometimes yelled incoherently at
me and then slammed down the receiver. Other
conversations were as if we had lived in a close
mother/daughter relationship. I went for a visit to*

see for myself and her blank eyes and gaunt appearance revealed more of the story. My three brothers met me for lunch and begged for my help. They didn't want her in a home, mostly because of money, I think, but they didn't want her at her home or their homes either. So I packed her a little bag of clothes, coaxed her into my car, and drove her back to my house.

She's not very happy with this arrangement and she constantly talks about going home. I just tell her we'll go home tomorrow and she is satisfied for a while. She can't go home. We sold her house and my brothers have lives of their own. But she is my mother no matter what and I will figure out how to get along and care for her as best I can. I am glad I have friends who listen to me and help me get through another day.

Nicole's love of her mom supersedes the pain of the past; her kind heart overrides the hurt. As a member of an Alzheimer's Support Group she can share her stress. With an Alzheimer's care grant she can get some in-home assistance. She is like many adult daughters. She has reversed the role of mother-cares-for-daughter (not very kindly, in Nicole's case) to daughter-cares-for-mother. Fortunately she has found some of the avenues of help.

Memory Activity #8 (page 151) in APPENDIX I *Healing: Writing and Reflection Activities* provides ideas for your writing for this section. Those with Alzheimer's, when life made sense every day, carried wonderful characteristics, characteristics that most likely also apply to you. Recalling relationships and friendships can help set your heart and your mind in motion for recovery.

There may also be difficult memories, ones that would be best erased. Confronting and rectifying the past may help eliminate some of the pain.

Notes and Reminders:

Chapter 9
Doctors, Hospitals, Medical Choices

Carole's Story

In her sixties and by then fully clutched by dementia, Carole had to face several operations. No longer the caregiver, she became the one to be cared for. The first operation was to remove bunions that appeared to be extremely painful because of their size. However, she bore pain under the double guise of Alzheimer's disease and quiet acceptance and so how much she hurt remains a mystery.

Carole headed off to the hospital fairly unaware of where she was going or why. Undressing her for surgery was a tussle as she fought people who were forcing her out of her clothes and into a ridiculous gown full of saggy, baggy openings and bothersome ties. Nurses and doctors are trained to take care of their patients, but often they do not understand that working with a person with Alzheimer's requires a different set of rules. Forcing Carole's clothes off and then forcing odd clothes on only resulted in increased fright and anger.

While we tried helplessly to intervene, "medical professionals" ignored us as uninformed, untrained, incapable outsiders. Simply saying, "Do you want to remove your shirt or your pants first?" or "Do you want this gown or that one?" would have eased the resentment and restored some dignity to Carole as she experienced a sense of control over the situation. Granted we had implemented this overbearing behavior in the past, forcing her into cars, into chairs, into showers, or into clothing but a step back and an offer of choice most often dissolved confrontation.

Post-surgery sedation and family patience allowed for ease of redressing and helping her climb into the wheelchair for the trip to the awaiting car and her return home. We had been warned to set up a bed for her in the living room and to purchase crutches for hobbling around the house as the doctor explained that she would be unable to walk without excruciating pain for days and maybe even weeks and that stairs would be a total impossibility for quite some time.

All of the best intentions of nurses, doctors, and other medical staff fell on deaf ears with Carole when we handed her the new pair of crutches. Unable to figure out how or why she should use them, she let them tumble to the ground as she wandered toward the front steps of the house and then ascended them effortlessly. Once inside we guided her to her new bed placed center-stage in the large parlor. With one disgusted glance at the "junk" in her living room, Carole resumed her wandering search: up the stairs, down the stairs, out to the garden and back. Pain did not exist for Carole even long after the painkiller effectiveness had vanished. Prowling was her lifestyle so she continued her rambling vigil.

Carole had two more surgeries during the final years of her life. The first was for a hysterectomy. While I do not think she really felt the pain from her condition and the surgery would not restore a fruitful life, doctors advised the procedure in case there was cancer developing. And so Rich followed doctor's orders and set her up for an operation.

Alzheimer's patients react differently to sedation: some go out like a light while others cannot reach adequate sedation. There is also debate about pain tolerance. Many do not seem to sense pain even when it would appear to be terrible like a burn from a hot stove or a broken bone from a fall. How Carole felt we do not know because she could not begin to tell us. She just rolled off to surgery and later returned with never a grimace or a complaint.

The real trauma from her second surgery began with the attending nurse after Carole was wheeled into her room and transferred to her bed. Although we had carefully requested that admissions write on her chart "Alzheimer's" and "Lactose intolerant" neither of these appeared to be noteworthy to the attendants in charge. Shortly after Carole settled into her bed, the nurse began her regular post-operation questions to check on her patient's mental state: "What year is this?" Silence. "Who is the president?" Silence. "What month is this?" Continuing silence.

The "What's your name?" silence broke the nurse. She huffed, rechecked the chart, scribbled scrawling notes, and mumbled something to us about, "We can't have this. She MUST respond." We offered a feeble explanation for Carole's confused silence but the nurse just muttered on about regulations as she stomped from the room with a hissed, "What are we to do?"

Carole had no inkling of who the president was. She did not even know her own name. Why did these silly questions even matter when an astute observer could recognize the veil of Alzheimer's that enveloped her? These routine and in Carole's case insensitive questions baffled her as they drove despair through us.

Later the same nurse returned to find that Carole had soiled the sheets. She reiterated, "We can't have this!" She then added, "If you pee the bed again I will put you in diapers!" With that thoughtless comment and conduct she exited.

We approached the bed and patted Carole's hand, reassuring her that everything would be all right. Carole stared blankly at us as one giant tear gathered at the corner of her eye and then slid down her cheek and tumbled onto the pillow. Fortunately, it was soon shift change and the inconsiderate nurse left us but not without resounding side effects.

Carole did not urinate again during her stay. Even though the staff plied her with milk (remember the lactose intolerance?) and other beverages, she refused to drink. I believe she was too scared and the nursing staff was too short handed to take the time to worry or care. They just wanted her to patch up quickly and go home, freeing the bed for someone else.

The final shock to the heart arrived when hospital officials handed Carole the release papers *(which she ignored) and they wondered aloud why she refused to sign her name. If she didn't even know her name, how could she sign it? Why would she even try? Neither my sister Jackie nor I had the authority to sign her release form either, so we awaited Rich's arrival to get her discharged and home from this nightmare hospital episode.*

Needless to say when Carole was sent home, hospital staff recommended bed rest with "no stairs or exertion". Deaf ears ignored this suggestion because she would not, could not obey the command so we also ignored it and let her do as she wished. You cannot force someone against his/her will and you definitely could not force Carole. Bed rest made absolutely no sense to her. Wandering around the house did and so her pacing pattern resumed.

Doctors, Hospitals, and Medical Decisions

Earlier I wrote about the doctor who ignored my mom because she was hard of hearing and she could not process his complete message. Even though her Alzheimer's disease was progressing she was still a thinking, feeling individual. The same was true of Carole. She may have been confused and lost, but she also had moments of cognition and awareness. I always remind my support group that the length of understanding disintegrates from hours to minutes to seconds but the seconds still count. They are tiny but important moments of connection, reconnection, and fragments of understanding.

Insight and Understanding

There is not knowing, not caring, and not wanting to learn or all of those bundled miscellaneously, haphazardly into most hospital stays. With an increase in longevity and the rising occurrence of Alzheimer's that comes with that, the medical world has much to learn about the care of those who cannot care for themselves. What if there is no one to speak up for and aid those who are surrounded by confusion? It is vital that you are prepared to ask for and demand appropriate care for your loved one.

I do not want to demean health care providers. There are wonderful individuals who seem to know intuitively the needs of someone with Alzheimer's; they understand the stresses of the Alzheimer's family. But there are also those who have no idea how to properly attend to some with this disease. Your background knowledge and experience play important roles even if you have to assert them to get others to listen.

Here are some tips to advance your knowledge of medical care concerns before, during, or after doctor visits, operations, and hospital stays:

- Select a qualified gerontologist, neurologist, and other health care professionals who are trained with the specific needs of those with Alzheimer's.
- Realize that over time medications and their effects on the individual change; discuss this with the doctor and your pharmacist. Visit websites that provide feedback on medical actions, interactions, and reactions such the Sanford Center for Aging at the University of Nevada Reno at www.unr.edu/sanford/programs/medtherapy.html
- Know that medications that work well with some patients may not work well with people with Alzheimer's.
- Maintain a journal of your loved one's changes in mental abilities and functioning to provide insight for care, medication, and interventions (before and after surgery; throughout everyday life).
- Even if you must address medical personnel with whispers, remind them that your loved one suffers from dementia but s/he is still a person who deserves kindness, patience, and dignity. Sometimes shouts are needed to produce necessary results but I recommend calm as often as possible.
- Sedation effects vary from no notable change to agitation, violence, and mounting confusion. Sometimes pain relievers work (or Alzheimer's disguises the pain) and sometimes they are ineffective. Every individual reacts differently. Watch, listen, note, and ask questions of others as they watch, note, and listen.
- Common devices like crutches or walkers can be mysterious and ineffective tools. Warn your physician that staying quiet and bed rest may be impossible to enforce with someone with Alzheimer's. S/he may

suggest restraints and that might work but I know I would suffer from heartbreak at the sight of my sister or mom bound to stop movement and prevent freedom (and dignity).

- No patient ever, regardless of medical condition, should be threatened over soiled sheets or not obeying "orders". Examination and evaluation of patient comprehension of hospital demands should be a top priority for you and your loved one. Accept that you may have to inform and educate medical personnel.

- Stay with your loved one if possible or tag-team the family for around-the-clock supervision while in the hospital. There are so many possible choices and decisions that may arise and untrained medical personnel may be at a loss as to a correct direction to take adding stress and confusion.

- Be aware that questions you can answer are not necessarily questions that the individual with Alzheimer's can respond to, right down to "What's your name?" or "Why are you in the hospital?" (routine medical questions at most facilities). Be prepared to answer for him/her if insensitive personnel persist with impossible questions.

- Even though hospital staff may be stressed and short-handed there is never a legitimate reason to treat any patient with anything less than dignity.

Reviving Hope

It is difficult to feel hope when you have been blown away by the behavior and actions of skilled medical professionals. It does not seem right that doctors and nurses who are trained to care for ill people could be heartless and uncaring. I have come to realize that most of these people really do care, but they lack the understanding and patience that are necessary when dealing with a hospital guest who has Alzheimer's disease. Practitioners who specialize in areas outside of elder care or dementia care frequently lack adequate training.

It thus becomes your job to offer and model some training to professionals who do not exhibit appropriate behavior. The note card again with:

112

Patience, please.

My loved one has Alzheimer's
works wonders in just about every situation. If this message produces no change or kindness effect, you may need to locate a new physician or facility.

If you are currently seeking a specialist contact your local Alzheimer's Association office for references and recommendations. There is generally a listing of physicians, facilities, in-home health care, and other agencies that specialize in dementia and elder care services.

Becoming Whole

There is a comical tale that goes along with the dreadful events just shared. Jackie and I stayed at the hospital with Carole during her hysterectomy. We found a tiny, lumpy rollaway bed for Jackie and I shoved two chairs together to create a makeshift bed for myself. The first night ticked by uneventfully. Carole slept and Jackie and I did the same. It was not a peaceful sleep under those odd bed conditions but we could not leave our sister alone in her lost world.

During the second night Jackie and I suffered from exhaustion resulting from our bedside stand. Carole had dozed in and out for most of the day and by night she was restless. We arose several times to calm and reassure her then drenched in darkness and silence we fell into deep sleep. Suddenly a jingling sound of sliding metal hooks and the clanging of an IV stand jolted us as light intermittently flashed into the room. Sliding to the floor in a snarl of tubes Carole had become entangled in the long privacy curtain and her IV. Wrapped like an odd shaped present, she struggled toward the door in her tangle and attempted to drag the curtain open.

Jackie and I zipped up, unraveled the curtain/tube/Carole mess, and guided her back to the bed, buzzing the nurses' station to report that she had been up and ready for a getaway. We prepared to throw ourselves on their mercy as inattentive caregivers if they would just help us soothe her back to sleep. No worry about chastisement as no one ever responded to our buzz. In fact nurses and doctors rarely stopped by to check on Carole. After all she never listened to or responded to them anyway so why try plus she had her sister guardians.

113

frustrations and false starts taught me that many who have never coped with Alzheimer's disease do not realize the significance of personal autonomy in one who appears unable to deal with current reality but who is still a person with needs and certain, though fading, abilities. Even in her darkest Alzheimer period Carole (and her sisters) needed and expected respect and dignity.

We were wrong to not intervene more vehemently on behalf of our sister. We tried to go long to get along. With what I now know, the indiscretions shown my sister will never occur in my presence again. I have learned to stand up for those who are unable to stand up for themselves.

Renewal Resources

There are many books and brochures to study before your loved one enters the hospital and there are many questions that you need to ask in advance. Take notes, ask more questions, take notes, and ask more questions. An elder care doctor will be prepared and ready to help you and the dementia patient. A doctor bent only on treating the problem and not on understanding the underlying worries of the individual with Alzheimer's and you and your family may not be the physician you want in charge.

Questions that you may have for the doctor:

- What do you know about and what are your experiences with patients with Alzheimer's and anesthesia? Recovery? Hospital stays?
- What side effects do the drugs you intend to administer or prescribe have for elderly patients and patients with dementia?
- What rehabilitation procedures will you recommend?
- How do I ensure that these procedures take place?
- What training can I receive in caring for my loved one after the hospital stay?
- How will you help me transition my loved one from hospital to home?
- What help is available for me when my loved one returns home?
- What is the prognosis for my loved one with the procedure? Without the procedure?

- What will health care providers cover and what will the family be required to pay?
- Is there equipment I can rent or purchases that will help me care for my loved when s/he returns home?

I'd really like to add, "Do you see my dear one as a person, a patient, a unique being or are you practicing medicine to practice?"

Also know that if the doctor and hospital tell you that your loved one is ready to go home but you sense that things are not quite right, that going home might produce problems, refuse the hasty exit. A dear friend was told her husband had to be "out by noon or else!" Marjorie, the caregiver, had heart problems, used a walker, and had uncontrollable shaking. Edward, her husband, had a difficult personality to deal with and he weighed more than 300 pounds. Does this sound like a reasonable release to home situation?

Memory Activity #9 (page 154) in APPENDIX I *Healing: Writing and Reflection Activities* offers suggestions for your writing for this section. Write, reflect, and share if you want to; guard your thoughts if necessary. Either method can bring you some peace.

The activities provided help you prepare for medical needs by preparing you to ask just the right questions and to ready you for a variety of eventualities.

Notes and Reminders:

Chapter 10:
Learning from Love, Dignity, and Alzheimer's
Writing for Me and for You

My Writing Story

So what finally triggered the inspiration for this writing? It was a Christmas cactus, the one that had decorated the funeral chapel and that I had received after Carole's service. Mine was a fuchsia explosion of blooming cactus. It was a lovely little plant, and I gently tucked it into our car for its trip from California to Nevada and its new home in my office.

While the memorial had been held on a balmy California "winter" day, the drive home was a snow-driven blizzard over Donner Summit and into Reno. Drifts were several feet high and blowing ever higher as we plowed down the freeway and exited onto north Virginia Street for the final ascent to our son Stan's home. A mound of fleece covered the street and we spun into an enormous drift and shimmied to a halt. We bundled into our coats and slipped out of the car to shovel and shove the car the last inches up the hill. It refused to budge. Failing forward progress, Stan gathered his bags from the trunk and began the trudge to his home, waving to us as he vanished into a blur of white.

Lynn, Allison, and I slid backwards down the hill until we could spin around and continue our snowy homeward journey. The wintry cold leaked into the car even with the heaters blasting. I glanced at the Christmas cactus cuddled in the back seat sheltered from a frosty death. Several hours of whiteout driving brought us to Winnemucca as the wind pushed us along and eventually dumped us into our driveway. Exhausted and bleary-eyed we emerged to more puffs of snow and icy cold. I wrapped the cactus under my coat to protect it from the pelting snow and I am certain I felt it tremble as I carried inside and settled the now slightly bedraggled pink and greenery onto its new perch on my desk.

I watered my cactus faithfully, supplied plant food as needed, and spoke to it softly, especially in the early morning as I set about my daily writing routine, but I did not really stop to listen to what it was attempting to whisper back to me. I did not pay attention to the tiny changes that brewed within it, to the message it was trying to convey.

Months melted away as did the snow as the cactus peered at me. It was not ever disdain or anger the cactus sent my way, but rather a tired sigh of resignation at being ripped from better climes to wait here in a room where quiet enveloped it and I ignored it. Oh, how powerfully the words *ignore* and *ignorance* are linked in meaning. It must have been simple ignorance that allowed me to ignore my precious gift for so long.

Spring arrived and then summer, and soon it was fall and winter again. The anniversary of Carole's death came and went and still the cactus lay in wait. Another year followed as my life rolled forward, wrapped in memories of Carole, but never memories that I could fully bring to the surface or put into print. There were shoots and starts for the cactus as new growth tipped the end of each branch and older branches fell, faded and dead, just as there were shoots and starts in my mind for writing about my sister, about my mom, about my experiences with Alzheimer's disease.

During this time the little cactus had near brushes with destruction. I had grown tired of the many plants I had cluttering the house. While some were beautiful many hung on to weak shreds of life. Between dying leaves and stems and leaky old, calcium-encrusted pots, I determined that it was time to clear out my plant menagerie. At the first sign of failing greens, I urged the plant's end along and then quickly and surreptitiously deposited it into the trash. Delivering each plant into the depths of the landfill was no easy decision. I always waited until Sunday evening or early dawn Monday, the last possible chance to extend their existence in my home before I slipped them out for the garbage collector so that they could quickly rumble away.

Over time the cactus began to appear frail and so one day I gathered the courage to dispose of it. It no longer was much of a looker having toppled off its perch on several occasions, crushing its branches and dumping its dirt. No one but me would have ever known it had been trashed. But my bravery began to wane as I glanced at it. I stared and studied finally recognizing its innocence; it was not yet time for the cactus to go to the dump. It still had a tale to tell. I knew it. I waited patiently and then one day it happened.

My cactus miraculously transformed from a mild-mannered houseplant into an explosion of cherry-pink blossoms. For this profusion there are two possible explanations. First, I offer the scientific one.

My family and I had exited frosty Winnemucca over spring break to soak in the radiating heat of Arizona. The house was locked up tight with the furnace turned down low and frigid air permeated every nook. While we basked in the sunny warmth of Phoenix, our town shivered with ice. Word is that Christmas cacti like to be removed from heat to spend time in extended cold. Enough cold after enough days and the plant forces its blooms. I guess the substantial days of cold created a blossoming condition in my plant and shortly after our return; tiny "budlettes" began to appear.

Initially they were minute dots at the end of each branch, looking more like errant ink spots than blossoms, but they were definitely a color splatter that stood out against an ever-more pronounced shimmering green. Little by little, day after day, the pink became brighter, bolder, bigger, and prouder. From dots and spots, to splashes and dashes, and finally to prolific explosions of glorious flowers, the Christmas cactus burst its feathery downs. Like single-colored pink peacock tails, they emerged on every branch of my plant. It no longer looked like a clump of unharmonious matter but like a vision of glory, vibrant with life. A scientific-minded gardener friend explained to me that the cold caused the blossoms to stress and bloom and fill my plant and my house with colorful wonder. It was as simple as that. That is the way of a Christmas cactus.

But there is a second version to the blossoming story, another possibility to explain the phenomenon. When we returned from vacation I knew in my heart it was time to write about Mama, Carole, and Alzheimer's disease; no more excuses or procrastination, just designated time for keyboard and me and a spill of words and emotions across the screen. Family had encouraged me, friends supported me, Carole and Mama beckoned me, and my support group cheered me forward.

On the day I spotted those first dots I thought perhaps my eyes were fooling me with floating specks. On second glance the dots grew clearer and I knew that something magnificent was simmering beneath the tip of each branch. I paused, drew in a deep breath, and stood in awe at such simple and perfect beauty. The buds transmitted a signal and reminded me of my promise, to write this deeply personal account of my journey and journal of lessons and learning of this devastating disease. It was time to gather the courage and set my brain on productivity mode, and tap my knowledge into print.

To organize my writing plan I donned my jogging gear and headed out for my long run, pounding out through my feet my thoughts of the cactus, its unique loveliness, and my Alzheimer's story. Miles thundered by and daylight began to break. The brightness of the dawn struck me with the real significance of this blooming day and my urgent responsibilities. Just one year ago to the day my father-in-law had died of MRSA. One moment Tommy was with us and within hours he had slipped into a coma and was gone. How could such a strong and innocent man be swallowed in one deep gulp?

As I ran my thoughts crystallized and I understood my responsibility. In the blaze of sunrise and through the cactus signals, Carole was sending me reassurance to prod me along. Somehow, in the mystery of life and death, Tommy, Mama, and Carole had joined together to push me to write this book.

Insight and Understanding

This awakening that nudged me to write about Alzheimer's has brought me to new understanding. It seems that the greatest learning often occurs from the lessons of the most profound aches of life. I share my hesitancy to write to let you know that reflection and putting ideas into written words has not been easy but it has been uplifting and gratifying as it fills me with a sense of renewal and a better appreciation of so many aspects of life.

One of the greatest fears of writers, a fear that fuels hesitancy, is getting the words and message right. And so as I write and re-write, edit and adjust, I admit to myself that this story will never quite reach perfection but it has already changed me and I believe that it may make a huge difference in the lives of many readers. That is powerful motivation.

With Alzheimer's disease, death is a slow, debilitating process. While it might seem like saying good-bye would be easier because there is plenty of time, time is never adequate. After a death and with time for reflection, rediscovering the goodness in life permits healing and growth. Sometimes the prompts for healing appear from unexpected and unlikely sources. Maybe you have a Christmas cactus in your life, a special indication reverberating in your direction as it attempts to guide you to insight and understanding. I promise you that writing really works! Writing empowers you as it clarifies vision of the past and vision for the future.

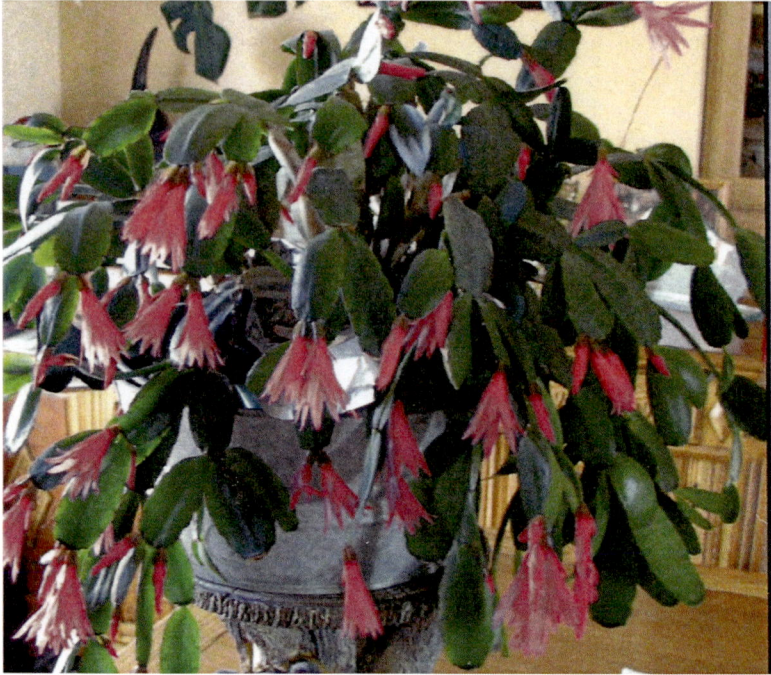

Reviving Hope

It is time to look around you as you learn to recognize the goodness of people and beauty of the world. My mom, sister, and support group have hopes to share with you:

- Teresa – *We were out to dinner the other night and Karl was acting nervous and agitated. Things were spilling (including my tears) when out of nowhere a rescuer appeared. He sopped up our mess, gathered to go boxes and put our meals in them, and then he gently urged Karl out of his* seat, out of the restaurant, and into the car. I was so thankful.

- Martin - This is supposed to be retirement and here I sit at home with Margaret who declines every day. I have been patient for 8 years but today I was set to explode. Then a knock came on the door and there stood my son and grandson. "Hey, Dad, how about some fishing? Giselle [daughter-in-law] will stay with Mom so you have no worries." I wonder how he knew, out of the blue, that I desperately needed this break?

- Marilyn - Frank fell out of bed and since he is a big man I could not get him up. I called 911 and the officer arrived in a flash. He helped me get Frank up before the paramedics arrived. Vital signs were wobbly but Frank refused an emergency room visit. The officer comforted me and said to just call when I needed his help. I needed it way too soon. The next day Frank fell again and almost before I dialed, help stood by my side. I am lucky to live in such a caring community.

- Barney - We had just sat down to breakfast when we noticed that Victoria had vanished. One minute she was tromping the kitchen, the next minute she was gone. We ran out the door and started hollering, running like crazy people. I headed down our road, calling all of the time and then I saw her, standing on the side of the road with two women. They smiled and calmed me, "She's fine, just a little lost. We saw her wandering and could tell by her eyes that something was missing, that something was lost." What handy helpers!

- Carmella - Jean-Marc and I first met when he vacationed in my village. I was fifty-two and he was seventy, but it was love at first sight. I had never married as I had cared for my elderly parents; his wife had died three years earlier. Two months later we were married and I returned home with him. We were so happy but

121

his daughters were not so happy. They saw me as a money-stealer instead of a woman who loved their father. They went to their attorney and made Pappi go along. They made sure everything, every decisions was in their hands and out of mine. They convinced Pappi that they could care for him far better than this foreign wife.

I love him, and I will stay by him, even as his mind fades. I am a good caregiver. The daughters would like to tuck him away in a facility, to take his home and property and sell them and divide the money between them. I don't care about the money. I care about Jean-Marc. I will keep him in our home as long as he wants to be here. When he is gone, I will figure out what to do next. The laws for a second wife can be troubling.

- *Thomas – I was in tears, my heart was breaking. My sister Annette had wandered off again and although I found her quickly, San Jose is a big city. Imagine what could have happened to her. In frustration I called our Alzheimer's hotline. As I shared my tale the dear person on the other end offered me support and options. She told me about the Alzheimer's Activity Center, a place of love and joy where Annette could spend the day busy with friends. I hung up relieved and then drove over to the center to see for myself. It has been a perfect choice.*

- *Jackie – Carole had been sinking and suffering and although I didn't want to, I decided it was time to allow her to go. I held her hand and whispered, "It's OK, Carole. I'll be all right. You can go now if you want to." And just like that Carole's breathing slowed to a raspy rattle. In shock I shouted, "Wait! I didn't mean right now!" Breathing resumed, she sort of smiled from the Alzheimer's haze, and she lived several more days. Never underestimate the power of words!*

- Kjelsey - *I was about five years old when Aunt Carole stopped by our farm on the way home from the cabin. While the family settled in for a game of cards, Aunt Carole appeared lost and bewildered. I snuggled up to her, then I grasped her hand and said, "Aunt Carole, come with me." I led her down the hall to my room where an enormous stack of dolls greeted us. "Let's play house!" I exclaimed and Carole joined right in. She was at ease touching my dolls, hugging them tenderly, and laughing with me. We made a connection that I will never forget.*

- Allison - *When I was three I loved the merry-go-round more than any other ride. The family was all at Great America and they took me on a few rides but then all refused one more merry-go-round whirl. Accept Aunt Carole. She climbed aboard and we rode for hours. Looking back I know she was lost in Alzheimer's at the time but she was still with me in a special way.*

- Gini - *When Mama moved to Weiser Alzheimer's grasped her but she still lived fairly independently. We thought it would be fun for her to ride the senior bus to the center for lunch each day, just to have a sense of purpose. The first couple of visits went all right, I guess, and then my sister got a phone call. "Your mom cannot make decisions on food and she is holding up the serving line. She cannot come back without supervision." Wasn't there someone amongst all of those seniors who would help, I wondered? It seemed odd to me that a senior center would reject a senior. Then Marlene stepped in to save the day. She offered to come to the house to have lunch with my mom. She even would have driven her to the senior center but I had hard feelings about that place so they established a lunch routine that lasted for a long time. Those lunches made Mama feel special.*

- Steven - *Magdelina and I had each lost spouses when we found each other. Her first husband had died of cancer; my wife had died from a long illness. We each know the agony of losing a loved one in slow, painful steps. We also recognize the benefits of continuing our lives after their deaths. The laughter and joy we share offer us safety and comfort that we could not have discovered in any other way. Just waking up every day with love and a purpose has added strength to our lives.*

Magdelina is in an early stage of Alzheimer's now, the forgetting and confusion stage. She has gotten short with the kids and grandkids but she still senses some remorse when she snaps. I don't like the idea of becoming a caregiver again, but then I have so many things to be thankful for including Magdelina.

- *Stan — I will never forget Carole's kind heart. She loved me in such a special way. One time I was chasing some geese on a sea-doo and she became so angry. I was far out on the lake but when I glanced toward the shore, I could see her shaking her fist and her mouth yelling words I could not hear. She was so upset. I made a promise then to never hurt my Aunt Carole again.*

  When she had one of her surgeries, I had just stepped onto the elevator to go see her when they rolled her gurney in the other door. She reached her hand out to me and she smiled. She recognized me even in the shade of Alzheimer's. I knew then that she had forgiven me.

- *Judy — When Carole was little she dreamed of a big, beautiful house with several children. She ended up with a lovely home and just one daughter. Carole became the epitome of the perfect Mom, so devoted and kind and caring. Every child deserves a mother like my sister. The world would be a happier place, I guarantee.*

Becoming Whole

Be on the lookout for special people and special moments. They exist everywhere although sometimes it may feel hard to locate them. Always remember that you do not need to travel the Alzheimer's journey alone. There are friends and organizations to help and comfort you. They offer safety and advice and they will listen to you.

Remember too that through the clouds of Alzheimer's disease, your loved one dwells within. Communication and interaction techniques from the past may now be useless, but the unique being still resides inside. Small, special moments of connectedness bring great (though temporary) joy as you learn to communicate in new forms.

Sometimes becoming a volunteer for a group can regenerate vitality in your life. I know it can be hard to imagine volunteering outside of your home when there are so many demands within it, but it just may work. There are organizations in every community that need you and your abundance of talents. Your goodness will boomerang back to you in infinite ways.

Renewal Resources
- The Alzheimer's Association – www.alz.org
- John's Hopkins University website on Alzheimer's and aging www.johnhopkinshealthalerts.com
- Elder care services of your town, city, and state (laws vary from state to state so check on the rules of your state)
- Elder care attorneys – these specialists will be familiar with laws that help you care for those who are unable to care for themselves (laws vary from state to state so check on the rules of your state)
- Elder care/geriatric physicians – medications that worked at 45 may have a quite different effect at 75. Physicians familiar with aging can provide you with essential health information
- Hospice – some groups work only with patients during the last months of life; others provide respite to caregivers in need regardless of the age or need of the victim. Check with organizations in your area that can help you or that need the help you can offer.

- Alzheimer's Support Groups – most communities have a group that meets at least once a month. Check the phone book or your state organization for more information. Sharing with and learning from others who face the Alzheimer's maze can be reassuring and very beneficial.

You are never alone. There are dear people to support you during the difficult, extended descent into Alzheimer's disease. Rest and care for caregivers are just as vital as care for individuals with Alzheimer's.

Memory Activity #10 (page 156) in APPENDIX I *Healing: Writing and Reflection Activities* steers your writing for this section. You are now a full-fledged, dedicated, proficient and prolific writer. Here is your chance to jot down your angel stories of people and things that have helped you on the Alzheimer's journey. Your insight and wisdom hold promise for opening and healing your heart and they may offer great security and understanding for others should you decide to share.

Notes and Reminders:

APPENDIX I
Healing: Reflection and Writing Activities

Clara's Story - Discovering Writing

John and I shared 54 years of marriage. We had raised seven children, held jobs we enjoyed, traveled, and loved deeply. Then Alzheimer's struck. At first John forgot his keys; then he forgot how to use money; then he forgot how to take part in his favorite hobbies. One by one he forgot the kids or mixed them with the grandkids. Finally he forgot me.

He forgot me but we still spent five more years together. I loved John for who he was and who he had been. I never considered skilled nursing although some of our children encouraged it and in hindsight, I would have had more patience and had a better outlook much of the time with some extra help. But even with the exhaustion of confusion and daily loss, I am glad I could care for John until the end.

The first months after John's death were a heart-wrenching blur. Right after the funeral family and friends called every day and I longed to be alone. Then the visits slowed and I found myself really alone for the first time in more than sixty years. It was awful. I ached, cried, and boiled with anger, but I always put on my happy face for others to see. They needed to know that I was fine.

Then one day I woke up and said to myself, "Enough!" I started writing about John, the good, the bad, the tough, and how he touched my life – still touches it today. Recovering from death is indescribable, painful, and dark. Family and friends help but much of it is a solitary journey. Emerging into the light again has breathed life into me. Writing has helped me reflect, remember, and live. I believe John would be happy for me.

Time, Reflection, and Writing Activities

The Memory Activity section is to support and guide your reflections and healing through writing. Some of the wondrous gifts of writing include:

- It is safe – Share with others if you feel you should; guard your thoughts close to your heart if you think you must.

- It is serene – There is power in words, power to make you stronger and wiser, but this power is also gentle. The words you select comfort you while clarifying your memories and understanding of personal loss.

- It is lasting – Written words are forever. Even if you maintain privacy throughout your writing, your words are here now and in the future. Your words are you on paper, are in print. They exist because you have created them and from this creation you have found rejuvenation.

- It is honest – While people blurt out lies for protection or to ward off the bad, you really cannot write lies to yourself. After all, you know the truth, all of the truth. Sometimes this truth has been hidden by memories, lack of clear understanding, and inexplicably painful reality, but it is there for you to find when you seek it. The truth of your writing is truth as you view it, as you live it. Truth is a powerful device.

- It is healing – Through the safe, serene, lasting honesty of words you will discover things about yourself that perhaps have never before been articulated. The more you write, the better you become at reflection. The better you are at reflection, the better you will know yourself. The better you understand yourself, the better you can deal with happiness, sorrow, and other truths of life. Writing is phenomenal.

Renewal Resources

Each activity reflects the key points of its corresponding chapter and is numbered accordingly. You may want to review the chapter before or during your writing.

You may just want to write. All activities are designed to help you heal with the powerful insight gained from uncovering your emotions and confronting loss. It is not simple to forget pain and move on, but dealing with heartache brings greater understanding of life.

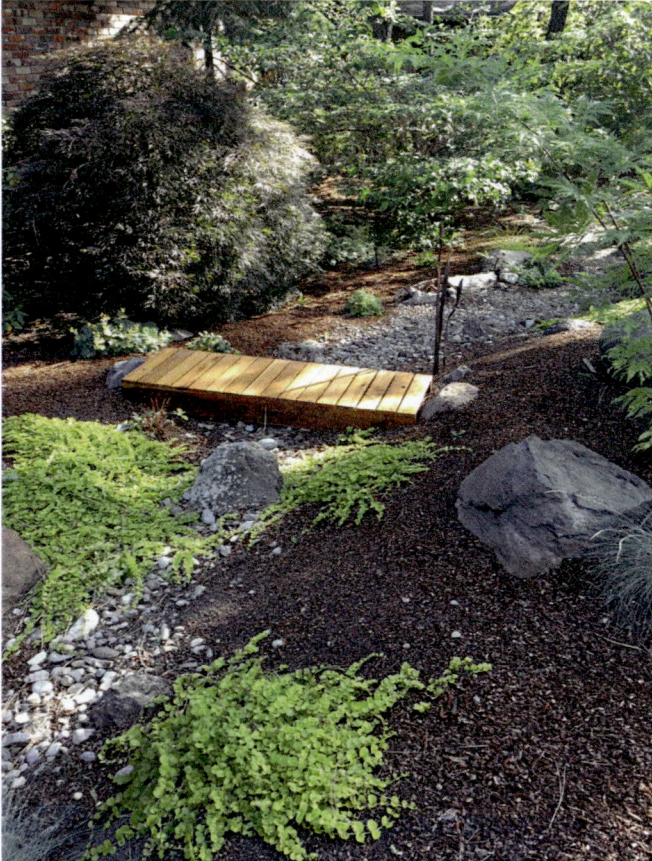

Memory Activities
Introduction Activity
Making Sense of No Sense

Healing takes time, requires distance from the pain, demands patience, and you must be persistence. Writing has the potential to channel your emotions and memories into serenity and the ability to live on, happily. Recall the earliest happy memory of the one you love. Describe what makes that memory so special.

Happy Memory

What are the special positive characteristics that you admire most about the one you love?

How are those characteristics reflected in you?

Recall a painful memory of the past. Determine three to five words that describe that pain. Confronting pain helps you overcome it and it helps move you toward healing.

1.
2.
3.
4.
5.

Recall a second happy memory. By balancing emotions with good/bad/good or happy/sad/happy, always beginning with a positive memory, alternating with a bad memory, and then ending with a positive memory, your mind gravitates to pleasant memories that settle on you and bring peace.

Happy Memory

List three to five words of happiness that come from this memory.

1.

2.

3.

4.

5.

Keep these words near your heart to support you as you heal.

The next activity helps you generate words that are personal and important to you.

Memory of_____

Happy Memory of _ _ _ _ _	Painful Memory of _ _ _ _ _
Adjectives to describe:	Adjectives to describe:
What I learned:	What I learned:

Key Word(s) and Sentence for _ _ _ _ _

Key word:
Key Sentence:
Defining sentence of _____:

Writing really can launch your insight to understanding. Everything truly does become clearer when put into words. Slowly and surely through determination and a belief in life and happiness beyond death a positive vision can return. While it may be difficult to begin with, know that you have the power to write; you have a story to tell that no one else can tell. Your words are valuable and essential for your healing and they may have a powerful impact on others if you want to share your thoughts and reflections.

Chapter 1: Memory Activity #1
Actions and Reactions; 10 Initial Warning Signs

In Chapter 1 *Actions and Reactions; Initial Warning Signs* you read about ten of the possible signals of the presence of Alzheimer's disease and other related dementias. Remember that these signs may indicate Alzheimer's but they may indicate a far different diagnosis. When you suspect a problem begin to document and journal about it: the changes, the worries, and the contradictions.

Signals	The Signs	Date(s)
1. Memory loss: forgetting recent information		
2. Difficulty performing familiar tasks: planning a day, following directions, using the phone		

Other symptoms...

3. Problems with language: finding the right word, making up stand-in words, confusing speech or writing		
4. Orientation to time and place: becoming lost, forgetting familiar locations		
5. Poor or decreased judgment: dressing inappropriately for weather, problems with finances		

6. Trouble with abstract reasoning: difficulties with complex tasks, forgetting how numbers work		

And then…

7. Misplacing things: putting things in unusual places		
8. Changes in mood or behavior: displaying sudden mood swings, agitation		
9. Changes in personality: becoming suspicious, confused, fearful, dependent		
10. Loss of initiative: becoming passive, disinterested, sleeping more than usual		

Modified from the warning signs of the Alzheimer's Association

Chapter 2: Memory Activity #2
Admitting a Problem, Receiving a Diagnosis
Traveling the Emotional Gambit

In Chapter 2 *Admitting a Problem, Receiving a Diagnosis; Traveling the Emotional Gambit,* we examined grief and its many manifestations. Unburying the truth of grief is complex because grief comes and goes, appearing and reappearing in new forms, guises, and disguises. Emotions are rarely simple.

Starting by examining what you are doing to maintain your health and then continue to the framework that reviews the nine emotions of grief and offers a guide to help you during and after loss as you move toward acceptance and wholeness.

My Health - How Am I taking Care of Myself?

Aspect of Health	Ways I take care of me so that I can better take care of _____.
Physical health	
Emotional Health	
Psychological Health	
Spiritual Health	

All emotions guide you in the direction of acceptance. Healing permits you to achieve a sense of safety and well being, even after the most tragic and traumatic events. A broken heart is never simple to repair.

135

Enduring Grief

Emotion	The event, the moment that best exemplifies the emotion	How I have (or will) learn to accept
Denial		
Admitting		
Anger		
Blame		
Helplessness		
Guilt		
Regret		
Forgiveness		
Acceptance		

Chapter 3: Memory Activity #3
Circuits that Are Not Circuitous
Navigating the Terrain

The following guide lists possible examples of forgetfulness, possible interventions, and then a space for you to record changes that you have noticed that might be signals and warnings that mental function is declining and that memory is not operating well.

Warning Signs of Problems
Problems, Concerns and Possible Remedies
Your Experiences

Problem	Concerns and Possible Remedies	Your experiences
Daily tasks	Getting up, selecting clothing, planning the day. Making and eating breakfast; sticking to a routine. Washing clothes, dishes, keeping house	
Knowing names	Recognizing family and friends and knowing their names and relationships; confusing father and son, grandson to uncle	
Knowing and recognizing places; following directions	Driving may be confusing, directions impossible; familiar places like the grocery store may just be a jumble of foods; cooking a familiar recipe may involve too many baffling steps to complete	

Eating properly	Check out Meals-on-Wheels or other food delivery service; take her out to eat; take her grocery shopping; encourage her to eat healthy snacks; always have a sandwich in a zip lock bag ready for her to eat	
Dressing properly	Selecting matching or appropriate clothing may be a problem, i.e., skirt and pants together, no coat in winter. Clean out closets and drawers so that choices are suitable and not overwhelming	
Too much time alone	Enjoy games, puzzles, mental stimuli; plan trips to the store, to concerts and plays; learn to avoid places that are too dark or too loud; enjoy hobbies and crafts that are fun and without pressure; share walks and talks; set up visits with family and friends; chat and listen	

Hygiene habits	Showers or baths, nail clippings, and getting clothes in the wash become problematic; purchase no tear shampoo; install a removable shower head; get rid of clothes that are holey or that no longer fit; purchase clothes that are bright, stylish, and easy to get on and off	
Conversing	Include the Alzheimer's victim in conversations as much as possible; the responses may not make sense but nods and reassurance can be powerful confidence builders; being left out is painful even though it may appear that the victim is entirely unaware of passing events	

And this may break your heart...

Getting along	Confusion, loud voices can make the victim feel under attack or as if others are ganging up in a negative way; outbursts may be wild and violent and no calming technique works. Change the subject or move victim away	

Seek diversions	Good senior centers offer activities, trips, and nutritious meals; attend events with the one who is loved; be certain that an angel takes your place when you must be gone	
House cleaning	Start from the beginning so piles of papers and bills do not accumulate; hire help for toilet and kitchen cleaning; extend duties to others as needed to rest caregiver and victim. Do not throw things away — just in case they are needed	

A tough decision...

Driving and transportation	Discontinue driving privileges when it is no longer safe — ouch! This is painful; contact OutReach or other means of transportation to get your loved one to appointments, etc.; off to drive the victim to appointments	

Dark places	Avoid them – they are scary. Dark carpet, dark closets, dark hallways, dark sidewalks – beware.	
Loud, blasting noises	Avoid them – they are scary. Loud conversations, games, songs, television – beware.	

It is sometimes difficult but...

Treat your loved one as an adult	Offer choices; be prepared for battles that make no sense; select battles that are worth the fight and toss aside those that only create frustration; never talk in his presence as if the victim does not exist	
Call for help	When others offer assistance, take them up on it; look for part-time help to give you a break; take care of yourself – caregiver respite is essential	

Look for Angels of Kindness and Goodness. They are everywhere! Often they appear at the precise moment when you are feeling the most desperate. It is amazing the marvelous work that an angel can do.

Be an angel to others. You will be rewarded many times over.

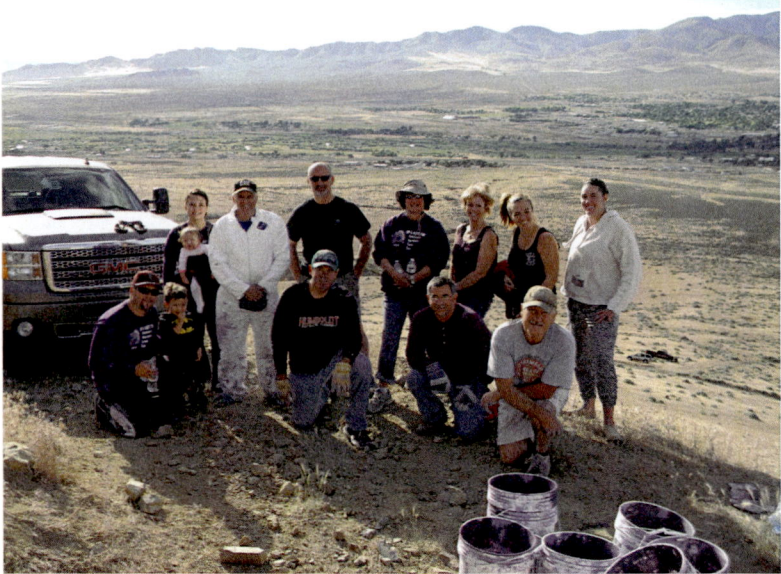

Winnemucca Alzheimer's Awareness Work Crew
Volunteers and volunteering are terrific!

Chapter 4: Memory Activity #4
Facing Baffling Reality
Family Diversity

Learning to provide choices makes such a difference in the happiness of a loved one with Alzheimer's. Small children like to feel as if they are in charge. "Do you want a green lollipop or a blue one?" Adults require the same degree of respect even when it feels as if they cannot choose or do not care.

Use the following diagram to examine tough decisions you may have to make or have made, searching for how each decision benefits you, your family, and your loved one.

Tough Decisions	Why this decision has/had to be made	The difference this decision made

Chapter 5: Memory Activity #5
Wandering, Searching, Losing the Way
Discovering New Paths

Readers who have loved someone dearly and lost him or her to any sort of death understand the agony of letting go. Those who have lost someone to Alzheimer's disease have a unique sense of the pain of losing someone over and over again. Reflect on your loved one as you complete the following activity:

Times Remembered

Time of Joy	What I learned	Time of Trial	How I Changed

Chapter 6: Memory Activity #6
Going Places, Eating Out
Remaining Connected

Think of several of the good deeds that your loved one has accomplished. Describe how two of these make you feel, even today. What have you learned as a result?

The Good Deed	How it makes me feel	What I have learned
Example: Carole loved animals of all varieties; her kindness rubbed off on me	Anytime I see an abandoned dog or cat, I move to the rescue as I know Carole would have done; it invokes tender emotions	Innocence comes in many forms, animal and human; love makes all things better

Now think about a bothersome event, one that made you question if anything in life would ever make sense again.

A bothersome time	How it makes me feel	What I have Learned
Example: When Candice came to our support group with bruises and tears	It made me feel ill to watch her anguish and to learn of her abusive spouse	I learned to listen, avoid judgment, and help Candice help herself

Notice how you are only allowed one bothersome event. That is not because there were not others, but rather that rough times bring us down and so does making them the focus of writing, reflection, and life. It is important to acknowledge that everything has not been, nor perhaps will it ever be, perfect. By concentrating on the positive but recognizing the negative, there is a range for reflection, growth, and healing.

There have also been angels along the way. Think about the kind people who have entered your life and how each one made living and life better.

Angels

Angel	When s/he arrived	How I was affected

Devils

Devil	When s/he arrived	How I was affected

There are many resources to support you during difficult times. Your phone book or an Internet search will help you locate some of these.

When friends offer to help, most often they mean it. Test them on the degree of their sincerity or amount of time they can devote by making simple requests – a loaf of bread from the store or a walk in the park. You do not have to take on every responsibility alone and those who love you want to help. Helping you helps them.

Chapter 7: Memory Activity #7
Personal Care
Maintaining Beauty

It is no simple task to move from being cared for to becoming the caregiver. Weigh what you can and cannot do for your loved one with Alzheimer's. Determine who is willing and able to help you and in what capacity. Consider whom you might hire to assist you.

Things I Need to Consider in My Care Plan

Clothing - easy on/easy off	
Shoes - good fit/consistent appearance to avoid unnecessary confusing	
Food - enough, easy to eat, easy to prepare; food allergies may develop	
Beverages - enough, easy to consume; straws and sippy cups	
Medicine - keep track of dosage and times to administer	

And what about...?

Personal hygiene - bathing and showers	
Bathroom needs - adult diapers, clean-up wipes	

Incontinence - am I prepared for this?	
Bathroom adjustments - rails, shower heads, grips	
Exercise - walking, light weights, stairs	
Mental stimulus - games, puzzles, conversations, socialization	
Emotional signals and changes - suspicion, anger, outbursts	
Housekeeping needs -	
Financial concerns -	
Bill paying needs -	

And just when you thought you were done...

Plans for travel - distance, sitting, bathrooms, changes of clothing, identification	
Facilities - unisex, cleanliness, large and open, light	

Nightlights, planning ahead for the dark, avoid confusing situations	

Special Caregiver Considerations

People I can count on to help me with these duties	
Things I want my loved one to know now	
Things other people should know	
Who to call on for help: family, friends, hotline, senior center, hospice	

Respite: How is the caregiver set to care for herself/himself?

Chapter 8: Memory Activity #8
Indecisive and Difficult Decisions
Seeking Peace

Think about your loved one's strongest characteristics and note how these strengths have carried over to you. Reflect on what you have learned from these characteristics. This reflection builds a brighter tomorrow when terrible memories are replaced with happy ones.

Name_____

Characteristic	How it is found in me	What I have learned as a result

And then there are all of those decisions and all of the people who have or want to have a say in those decisions. Carefully chart your course so that you will be ready with answers when questions arise about care for an Alzheimer's victim.

Weighty Decisions

Decision	What I think is right	What loved one has wants	Family sug-gestions	The Best Choice
No additional help or care				

Spouse, children or others attend to care				
Hourly care, 1-7 days per week				
Full day care: in-home or activity center/daycare				
Move to a locale closer to family				
Independent living with supervision				
Assisted living				
Long-term/ Skilled nursing				

Live with children				
Medical considerations				
End of life decisions				
Family diversity on decisions				

Other considerations:

Chapter 9: Memory Activity #9
Doctors, Hospitals, and Medical Choices

Many decisions arise when caring for a victim of Alzheimer's disease. A family doctor can be wonderful help, if he is up-to-date with caring for the elderly or those with dementia. Some doctors are happy to just give you some medicine or anti-depressants and send you home. You want a doctor who completes an initial, thorough exam that may rule out things like a urinary tract infection or anxiety as the cause for forgetfulness and disorientation. Then she requests a complete evaluation from a neurologist who specializes in the elderly and/or dementia.

On your visits be sure to bring your journal with all of the changes you have noticed in your loved one.

Journaling ideas

Changes in:

Mental outlook	
Attitude toward family and friends	
Attitude at work	

Personal worries...

Ability to complete job	
Hygiene and personal care	

Dressing	
Temperament	
Socialization skills (going out/interacting with others)	

Considerations for Medication or Hospitalization

Concern	Information/Solutions
Type of anesthesia to be administered	
Type of pain relievers to be administered	
Is the unit one that regularly deals with Alzheimer's patients?	
May I stay with my loved one?	
What in-home care can be provided after s/he returns home?	
Are there other alternatives to surgery?	
How will this surgery affect quality of life in the long-term?	
What should I expect when my loved one returns home?	
What physical therapy/rehabilitation is available?	

Chapter 10: Memory Activity #10
Learning from Love, Dignity, and Alzheimer's:
Writing for Me and for You

Select a memory that best matches your mindset and beliefs at this moment concerning the one you love. Begin by:

- Creating an image of joy that surrounds your loved one.
- Describing the feelings and emotions that that memory elicits.
- Searching for small miracles that signal the love of your dear one:
    - Coins left in just the right spot
    - Rainbows that arch across the sky when you least expect them
    - Wagging dog tails, purring cats, whirling snowflakes, laughing children
    - A tender phone call, email, or letter from someone you care about
    - Warm sunlight pouring in through your windows with beams warming your soul
    - Messages and gentle words seemingly out of nowhere that exude care and love
    - Blooming flowers, splashes of greenery, sudden explosions of color

Memory:
Key details:
How this memory helps me feel comforted and safe:
How knowing & loving this person has made better:

Angels may be at the heart of a place that you go to find peace, solace, and the beauty of the moment. It may just be a lovely day that enfolds you to make you feel just a tiny bit safer and stronger. Jot these Angel stories into your log. Think of ways to repay the kindness to others in need. There is enormous healing that comes when you are helping others as you are helping yourself.

Your Angel Events	How it made me feel:	How this act of kindness made a difference:

Final Thoughts...

For four years my mother melted away. For fourteen years I watched as my sister encountered the same fate. In both cases I knew they were "in there", just as I knew that they were less and less able to come out to interact with the world, even for an instant. With both of these loved ones I traveled the gambit of emotions. I suffered, I learned, I readjusted my thinking, and I ended up being a better, kinder, more conscientious person. Denial was a friend that allowed me to repeat to myself that nothing was seriously wrong.

Denial protected me, insulated me, and sheltered me from fear until denial became impossible and dangerous. I knew that forgetting occasionally is normal; forgetting constantly is not. To continue in denial meant I also risked the safety of Mama and Carole and intervention for them as well. While twenty-four years ago no doctors offered any medications for my mom, Carole took some that appeared to make a positive difference for her mental capacity and our peace of mind. And now there is even more hope for dignifying the lives and extending mental capabilities of people with Alzheimer's.

Eventually I forced myself to admit the presence of the Alzheimer's monster. I had no choice. In some ways admitting it felt like submission to the disease, but I know that by confronting it, truth and reality could step in to clear my vision and help me plan for the future. Admitting the presence of Alzheimer's did not necessarily mean accepting it; I believe acceptance came after death when fighting back had no result, when my survival and positive state of mind depended upon wisps of hope.

My mom and sister taught me again and again the significance of true love. Even when they could no longer express their tender caring in comprehensible ways, I know that they loved me, and more importantly, they both knew that I loved them. That knowledge provides me with strength and goodness. They taught me ways to make a difference in the lives of others through writing, listening, and volunteering. Our journey (and journal) is marked with lessons and learning.

Marilyn's story - Stitches

My first memory of life with Carole comes from when I was three years old; my sister Carole was eighteen months. I remember that Mama and Daddy were in the kitchen preparing for a day outing and Carole and I were standing between the dining room and living room sticking our fingers through the back of the door. When we became bored with that we took our play to a higher level. I stuck my tongue through the crack in the back of the door and Carole shut it. Blood spurted, I screamed, Carole cried, and Mama and Daddy came running.

The plans for the day were cancelled when I was rushed to Dr. Peterson's office on the Northwest Boulevard with a bleeding tongue. I received 5 stitches in the fleshy part of my tongue. My swollen tongue ached for weeks afterwards and it still bears the scar.

While Marilyn's scar is visible to remind her of this crazy game, we all carry the hidden scars from the sadness and loss. As I look back to when Mama and Carole were cognizant I wish I had said so many words of love, I wish I had asked so many questions about their lives. Then maybe I would better understand the internal pain and worry that Alzheimer's disease brought to them. I would have had more knowledge to help them and others instead of relying on memories and hindsight.

Some of these questions might have been:

- What worries do you have about your memory?
- How can I help you remember things?
  - A special calendar
  - Phone calls on certain days at certain times
  - An alarm or signal
  - Personal intervention...
  - Special in-home care
- What are some trips you would like to make, places you would like to go, things you would like to see or do to fulfill the wishes of your life?
- How can I best take care of you now?
- How can I best take care of you in the future?

- Will you please tell me one more story or your life? Your dreams? Your greatest accomplishments? The things that you wish you had done differently?
- Do you have final, end-of-life wishes of which I should be aware?
- Are you willing to share these with me?

We each grieve differently when we lose someone we love. Some people pick up and move on with barely any looking back. Others hurt so intensely that life becomes an impossible blockade against renewal. For me loss has compelled me to recognize the interconnectedness of our family and how our rich relationships have led me to this point in my life. I am so blessed to belong to a family who genuinely loves and respects one another. The significance of their impact on my life is profound.

Do I worry about having/getting Alzheimer's? Yes. It is not that I worry constantly but I do wonder every time I forget something like a name, a word, a place, or how to complete a task. Mostly I worry about the terrible burden that Alzheimer's heaps onto family and caregivers. I cannot fathom changing from the role of caregiver to my spouse and children to becoming the recipient of their care.

One day I shared with my daughter Allison my fear of the disease. What if the empty eyes and blank stare of my mom and sister transfer to me? My request was that if she recognized a spiraling mental decline in me with no hope of rising again, that she would take me out in a boat on a still Priest Lake morning and nudge me gently off the edge and into the cool, enveloping water. My dear-heart daughter burst into tears at this thought, a thought that peacefully soothed me as it terrified her. I then tried my oldest son who became equally upset at my request. My middle son I would not even ask - he is far to tender.

What would I do?

Many people approach me with questions about Alzheimer's disease. My experiences with Mama and Carole have educated me; my support group has added more background knowledge. Reading, research, and my regional Alzheimer's Association constantly advance my understanding. My monthly newspaper article, "Love, Dignity, and Alzheimer's" has spoken to many in my community. Some email me; others come to the support group meeting for discussion and information. A third group spots me in the store or at the post office and as they approach me, I sense their fear and anguish as they radiate from them. Alzheimer's is a terrible disease to contemplate, to recognize in one's life and in the lives of others.

When this last group speaks to me, it is invariably at close range, with direct, sad eye contact, and it always comes out in a whisper: *Thanks. We were wondering... The doctor says... Where should we turn to next?* I feel fortunate that these people trust me with this heartbreaking secret. It pains me that I cannot wave a wand and fix it all in a flash. I hope that someday in the near future that a magical wand will exist to wipe away the dread and horror of this intrepid disease so that no one ever again has to travel its cloudy, painful, and difficult road. Until then we can only hope.

SPINES - the 6 Keys to Maintaining Good Health

Key	Description
Social	Interacting with others: attending events, joining a club or activity group, and staying active and connected, volunteering...
Physical	Exercising every day whether walking, jogging, swimming, going to an exercise class, participating in yoga...
Intellectual	Working your brain: reading, writing, solving problems, completing puzzles, and actively engaging your brain...

Nutritional	Eating well: enjoy fresh fruits and vegetables, whole grains, lean meat, and dairy products; nutritional beverages...
Emotional	Keeping a positive outlook with worries at a minimum and stress at a distance; cry/laugh/cheer/scream as needed for balance...
Spiritual	Meditating or attending church services: finding peace and comfort in quiet reflection and stillness, renewing your being, refreshing your soul...

So How Do You Maintain Your Health?

Key	My Activities	Activities for My Loved One
Social		
Physical		
Intellectual		
Nutritional		
Emotional		
Spiritual		

APPENDIX II
Tips from Caregivers

I have been a facilitator for the local Alzheimer's Support Group for the past eight years. Each month we meet and talk. Sometimes we have a planned program or presentation. At other times we just share, support, and remind each other that we are a team who cares. They have taught me so much and especially that no one must ever travel this long, treacherous, unpredictable journey alone. This group generated the following tips to help you.

- Never argue – you cannot win. Just politely agree or redirect the conversation and move on.
- When the same problem or question reappears, agree, redirect, and move on.
- Deal with problems without being negative.
- Learn to go along to avoid anger and confusion.
- Redirect attention in positive, affirming ways.
- Agitation happens, especially with change. Display calmness so that peace can return.
- When agitation occurs, examine the situation to determine the cause so that you can avoid the situation in the future.
- Admit that there is a problem and know that there is help.
- Consistency is inconsistent – every day is new.
- Disturbances arrive "out of a blue moon". There might be environmental changes, perception changes, physical or mental decline, or something that cannot be defined. With time most of these melt away.
- Without diagnosis and doctor's advice, the early stages of the disease can be frustrating and confusing, especially for spouses and family. Since Alzheimer's is an "in and out and in again" disease it is hard to pinpoint exactly what the problem is.
- People with Alzheimer's in the early stages are good at masking a problem by avoiding bothersome situations. Their arguing that "everything is all right" can be easy to accept instead of seeking the truth.

- Verify that your physician understands problems of aging; if she does not, locate a neurologist or elder care specialist who does.
- Make an appointment with a neurologist who is trained in dementia and Alzheimer's for a thorough examination and diagnosis.
- Ask lots of questions; ask for an extended appointment time so that your questions have time for thoughtful responses.
- Check medications. As people age, medications react differently. It may be time for an adjustment.
- Check medication interaction. Most doctors say that if you are taking 5 or more medications, whether they are prescription or over-the-counter, each interferes with the effectiveness of the others.
- Forgetfulness has many causes besides Alzheimer's so a proper diagnosis is important. Poor nutrition, infections, stress, depression, or medication reactions are just a few possibilities.
- Be concerned about a doctor who in a casual glance concludes "Alzheimer's" without factoring the possibility of other potential problems.
- Patience – patience – and more patience. You cannot make sense of no sense.
- Caregivers need to take care of themselves; it is easy to think you can handle it all but burnout is a frightening sentinel.
- Continue to do activities together, just know that adjustments may be required.
- Avoid dark places with loud noises.
- Have family gatherings earlier in the day when it is light and bright.
- Avoid too much confusion. Maybe celebrate a birthday in small increments of people rather than a big, noisy bash.
- Repetition is repetition is repetition. Nod and move on. The victim is unaware of what has been said and so he may repeat it over and over.
- Caregivers need to do things independently at times for peace and for health.

- Interact with the victim with puzzles, activities, sorting clothes, building models, and conversing as if everything makes perfect sense.
- Remember what the victim formerly loved to do and tie it into activities of today.
- Small doses of activity work best as attention and interest span wane.
- Do not fight food issues. A healthy diet is important but arguments over it are not. Finger foods, sandwiches divided into quarters, small bites help increase food intake.
- If your loved one only eats ice cream, I think it is OK.
- Many older individuals develop allergies to foods like dairy products. Talk with your doctor if you notice some digestive problems.
- Drinking straws can be helpful in getting liquids into someone. Later the sucking reflex disappears so use a cup with a drinking spout to avoid spills.
- Strange fears arise in people with Alzheimer's but often there is a reason — dark rugs look like holes, black dishes appear unhealthy, loud noises sound like threats...
- Showers and baths can become frightening with clothes off, water dripping, and personal privacy invaded. Patience, gentleness, and accepting slow progress in the cleansing process are important.
- Personal hygiene may be forgotten, especially if the Alzheimer's victim lives alone. You may have to begin washing clothes, taking your loved one to a barber or beauty shop, seeking help from in-home health care services.
- Preparing meals can be confusing. Assist in preparing a meal and then sit down and enjoy it with the patient. A friendly voice and conversation have great positive effects.
- Deciding what to wear can become difficult. Put soiled clothes out of sight and set a choice of clothing on the bed or in the bathroom. If your loved one chooses something that does not match, who cares? If she chooses a swimming suit for the

snow, try to redirect toward something warmer but if you are staying in, avoiding an argument is wise.

- Select clothing that is easy on and easy off – snaps, ties, elastic, and loose collars are a good idea.
- Offer choices when possible. People with Alzheimer's are adults and they deserve respectful treatment. There are glimmers of thinking even from lost depths.
- There are good days and bad days, good moments and bad moments. The only thing you can count on is the constancy of change. But when it comes to remembering, head toward the good memories.
- Some individuals with Alzheimer's are very good at hiding or disguising problems by denying them, by refusing to address them, or by arguing so that caregivers will just back off. Again, reach into your bottomless bag of patience to figure out solutions without frustration.
- Law enforcement agencies can be helpful in returning wanderers or helping caregivers if violence erupts. Contact your local agency with your concerns and worries.
- Law enforcement agencies can be helpful in removing driving privileges. Taking away the independence of a loved one is not easy so it is nice to have a support team like the police to back this decision.
- Identification bracelets, watches, necklaces, or even peel-off sticky notes discretely placed on the back with a name and address can help if your loved one should wander away.
- Seek legal advice for items like Power of Medical Attorney, Power of Finances, Living Wills, Medicare and Medicaid. States have different requirements, forms, and procedures so be sure to check on your rights and responsibilities.
- Social workers and other social services can be helpful with advice on medical equipment and the correct level of care at a price that works into the victim's budget.
- Touch is healing – pats, hugs, tender caresses soothe.
- A tap or a gentle nudge can help get things rolling in the right direction or when redirection is

necessary. Gentleness is very important as force can create big problems.

- Love counts.
- Dignity is essential.
- Take time for yourself: a stroll, a night out, a trip to visit old friends.
- Volunteer to help others in little ways that reward you and that do not overwhelm you.

APPENDIX III

Caregivers Bill of Rights

Caregivers have the right to:

- Seek help.
- Receive support.
- Be angry and irritated.
- Take time to be alone.
- Request assistance.
- Decline assistance (even when it is in the caregiver's best interest).
- Trust one's own judgment.
- Acknowledge and address one's limits.
- Make mistakes.
- Grieve.
- Laugh and love.
- Maintain one's own active life.
- Reject attempts by relatives and friends to interject.
- Be granted consideration, affection, forgiveness, and acceptance.
- Expect that as new strides are made in finding resources to aid physically and mentally impaired individuals, similar strides will be made toward aiding and supporting caregivers.

Person with Alzheimer's Disease
or Other Dementias
Bill of Rights

Individuals with Alzheimer's have the right to:

- Seek help.
- Receive support.
- Be angry and irritated.
- Take time to be alone.
- Request assistance.
- Decline assistance (even when it is in the person's best interest).
- Remain independent unless this independence leads to eminent danger.
- Trust one's own judgment.
- Acknowledge and address one's strengths and limitations.
- Make mistakes.
- Grieve.
- Laugh and love.
- Maintain one's own active life.
- Reject attempts by relatives and friends to interject too many opinions.
- Be granted consideration, affection, forgiveness, and acceptance.
- Expect that as new strides are made in finding resources to aid physically and mentally impaired individuals, similar strides will be made toward aiding and supporting those with Alzheimer's and other dementias.

APPENDIX IV
Guidelines
Police, Highway Patrol, First Responders
Assisted Living Personnel and Caregivers
Medical Practitioners and You!

- Approach from the front, not from behind, to avoid startling or scaring the individual with Alzheimer's disease or other dementias.

- Speak calmly and evenly. Do not shout or appear aggressive

- Ask how you can help the person – he or she may be able to state that s/he is lost, scared, confused, cold, etc.

- If s/he cannot answer, check to see if the individual has an identification bracelet or GPS locator so that you can get more information about the individual and secure help.

- Do not argue or raise your voice. Combatant behavior leads to increased agitation and potential aggression.

- Nod and agree, even if the individual makes little or no sense, as you work to discern the problem and to find a solution.

- If a crime is involved like shoplifting, realize that an individual with Alzheimer's disease or other dementias probably does not understand this. S/he may lie, try to run, look wild, throw a tantrum, or cry. Stay calm, study the demeanor and the eyes, and avoid confrontation as you wait for help or for a family member to come to help you.

- Study the eyes. Individuals with Alzheimer's disease often have blank stares, an emptiness in the eyes.

- Those with Alzheimer's can be wily and explain one idea with clarity and the next with mixed confusion.

- If the individual is a wanderer, chat with family members about GPS or identification bracelet. Know routines so if the person wanders again, you'll be there to help.

- Someone with Alzheimer's probably cannot complete a multi-step process so avoid confusing instructions or items to complete in a series.

APPENDIX V
Risk Factors and other Information

- Age
- Genetic Mutations
- Family History
- Mild Cognitive Impairment — measurable changes in thinking abilities but these do not affect the individual's ability to carry out daily activities
- Cardiovascular Disease — the health of the brain is related to the overall health of the heart
- Traumatic Brain Injury (There is often a combination of these factors).

Beneficial Actions
- Education — building a cognitive reserve through higher education
- Social and Cognitive Engagement support brain health
- Exercise and Eat Healthy Food

Diagnosis
Primary Care Physician and Trained Gerontologist or Neurologist
- Examine medical records
- Ask family members about changes in thinking skills or behavior
- Seeking input from a specialist
- Conducting cognitive testing and physical and neurological examinations
- Having the individual undergo a MRI to identify brain changes, such as a tumor, that might explain symptoms

Alzheimer's Disease and Dementia
Caregiving Tasks

- Help with instrumental activities of daily life such as household chores, preparing meals, providing transportation, arranging doctor's appointments

- Helping with medications

- Helping patient adhere to treatment recommendations

- Assisting with personal activities of daily living such as bathing, dressing, grooming, feeding, and helping the person walk, transfer from bed to chair, use the toilet, manage incontinence

- Managing behavioral symptoms such as aggression, wandering, depressive moods, agitation, anxiety, repetitive activity, nighttime disturbances

- Finding and using support services

- Making arrangements for [aid in-home, nursing, and assisted living services

- Hiring and supervising others to provide care

- Providing overall management throughout the day

- Addressing family issues relating to caring for a relative with Alzheimer's disease including communicating with other family members about care plans and other decisions

APPENDIX VI
Recommended Readings and Resources

Each individual with Alzheimer's is unique. The disease manifests itself in a variety of forms and fashions. Sometimes the brain invasion is obvious as in juice poured on pancakes or being lost in the airport with dim eyes that reflect only confusion. Other clues are far subtler in their disguise such as forgotten names or misplaced car keys. It is the constant repetition of forgetting that may signal an alarm.

Some people with Alzheimer's are angry. They lash out over the least bit of change as every movement becomes a misunderstanding. Others remain calmly packed into memory loss, perhaps too afraid to even acknowledge the change, perhaps so entangled in forgetfulness that full awareness of the change is non-existent. Regardless of the situation, the slow descent is cruel and agonizing for family who is forced to look on helplessly for months and years and sometimes even decades as the disease destroys all bits of independence and ability. I can only imagine the terror that the loved one must feel.

As recommended throughout the book, one way to help in wading through and recovering from (caregivers and family) Alzheimer's is through writing: daily reflections, a journal, notes on passing events, or completing the activities in APPENDIX I Healing – Reflection and Writing Activities.

Although no cure is in sight and medicines offer only temporary masking of symptoms, a topic as enormous as Alzheimer's disease is rich with resources. Researchers express hope that even though there are limited possibilities now, there are enormous possibilities in the future. The following are books, hotlines, and websites that I have found to be beneficial to the understanding and increased knowledge of Alzheimer's disease.

Albom, Mitch. *For One More Day*. New York: Hyperion, 2006 Albom's book explores the regrets of the main character, Charley, as he relives his life searching for peace and understanding. This is a great resource for looking back and creating meaning in one's life and determining ways to make a positive impact by repairing past mistakes.

Alzheimer's Association — www.alz.org 1-800-272-3900
The website is rich with information and many downloadable
tools. There are also phone numbers for local and national
Alzheimer's organizations. Any time I have called, angels
answer with help and support.

Check on-line and in the phone book for local services such
as Alzheimer's support groups, hospice organizations, senior
centers, or dementia/elder care activity groups.

Callone, Patricia R. MA, MRE. et al. *A Caregivers Guide to
Alzheimer's Disease — 300 Tips for Making Life Easier.* New
York: Demos   Medical Publishing, LLC, 2006.
Caregivers need help and support and this book provides
many practical ways to care for yourself so that you can
better care for a loved one. Caregiver burn-out is
frighteningly real.

Cooney, Eleanor. *Death in Slow Motion. — My Mother's Descent
into   Alzheimer's.* New York: HarperCollins Publishers, 2003.
The title of this book expresses the essence of the entire
book. Alzheimer's disease is not sudden; it is a creeping,
crawly disease that robs its victim bit by bit until only a
shell remains. This thoughtful reflection supports readers as
they search for understanding and ways to deal with on-
going loss.

Dean, Debra. *The Madonnas of Leningrad.* New York: Harper
        Perennial, 2006.
Marina, the main character, lives in the present with
Alzheimer's disease nipping at her heals as she winds back
to the past and her days in the museum of Leningrad. This
back and forth life journey exemplifies for readers the
vacillating tendencies of Alzheimer's — it's here, it's not
here; my past ties to the present, my past is a mystery.
Understanding our parents and relatives helps us understand
who we are and this book creates a wonderful platform for
increasing inner exploration based on family past.

Diamond, Marian, PhD. and Janet Hopson. *Magic Tress of the
Mind: How to Nurture Your Child's Intelligence, Creativity,*

and   *Health Emotions from Birth through Adolescence.* New York: A Plume Book, 1998.
The title may seem out of place but it blends perfectly with Alzheimer's disease as brain development, intelligence, and creativity are plucked away one by one as the victim moves in reverse from active, vibrant adult to helpless, dependent infant. Ideas for activities and stimulation fill the pages.

Geist, Mary Ellen. *Measures of the Heart – A Father's Alzheimer's, a Daughter's Return.* New York: Springboard Press, 2008.
The author left her career to help her mother take care of her father as he fell into the dark abyss of Alzheimer's disease. Warmth and humor inspire readers with advice and support for helping those with the disease and also taking care of themselves.

Genova, Lisa. *Still Alice.* New York: Gallery Books, 2009.
This book focuses on a rare form of Alzheimer's that is not only younger onset but also advances with amazing rapidity. It is a tender story about a university professor as she plunges into the depths of Alzheimer's. The movie of the same name is also very good.

Whouley, Kate. *Remembering the Music, Forgetting the Words.* Boston: Beacon Press, 2011.
Based on the author's life spent caring for her mother, this book is informative and deeply moving. Whouley recounts the many struggles she faced as you wandered this disesae making critical decisions for her mother's life and well-being. Whouley is not afraid to discuss difficult topics.

The movie *Alive Inside, 2014*
    This film chronicles the research and action of Dan Cohen as he brings Music and Memory to care facilities across the nation demonstrating that music can transform a life. www.musicandmemory.org

Acknowledgements

The Alzheimer's disease stories of my mom, my sister, and my support group members have been distilling for many years. While it has been difficult to recall and then write about these complicated memories, it has also been rewarding and has provided me with wisdom, wisdom that I wish to use to help others.

I especially want to thank the following individuals:

My darling Mama who has shaped my life in so many wonderful ways

My dear sister Carole who suffered the Alzheimer's decline for fourteen long, torturous years

Could I have ever learned all I know about this disease without them to guide and motivate my writing?

My brother-in-law Rich: The most astounding, generous, and patient caregiver I have ever known.

My niece Karen, Carole's daughter:
In the web of loss one name remained in Carole's vocabulary – "Karen".

My sisters Marilyn, Judy, and Jackie:
We are so fortunate to have one another. Sisters are truly a gift.

My husband and children Lynn, TW, Stan, and Allison:
Your love of my sister and of me enlightens my writing.

The darlings of my Alzheimer's Support Group:
You empower me at each meeting with your stories and honest desire to be excellent caregivers and to reach out to others in need.

The Humboldt County Volunteer Hospice – Sherry, Sherry, and Cindy

May Love, Dignity, and Alzheimer's
A Journal of Lessons and Learning
provide you with the support and information
you need as you travel the twists and turns of this
relentless disease.

Please contact me with questions and to share your insight:

gini.cunningham25@gmail.com

Made in the USA
Middletown, DE
12 September 2015